HERBS FOR
HOME TREATMENT

HERBS FOR HOME TREATMENT

A guide to using herbs for first aid
and common health problems

Anna Newton

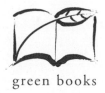

green books

First published in 2009 by

Green Books
Foxhole, Dartington
Totnes, Devon TQ9 6EB
www.greenbooks.co.uk

Design by Stephen Prior

Photographs © Anna Newton
and Neil Clarke LRPS

Printed in the UK by TJ International, Padstow,
Cornwall, UK. The text paper is made from 100%
recycled post-consumer waste, and the covers from
75% recycled material.

DISCLAIMER: This book is intended as an informational
guide. The remedies, approaches and techniques
described herein are meant to supplement, not to be a
substitute for, professional medical care or treatment.
They should not be used to treat a serious ailment
without prior consultation with a qualified health-care
professional. Neither the publisher nor the author
assumes any liability for any injury or damage to
person or property arising from this publication.

ISBN 978 1 900322 42 3

Contents

Introduction   8

PART ONE: OPTING FOR HERBS

Chapter 1 Why herbs?   11

Chapter 2 How to get the best from this book   15

Chapter 3 General precautions   16

Chapter 4 Herbs and the environment   18

Chapter 5 Tea, tincture or tablets?   21

Chapter 6 Dosage   25

Chapter 7 Choosing the right herbs for the situation   28

Chapter 8 How to combine herbs   30

Chapter 9 What if it doesn't work?   32

PART TWO: AILMENTS AND TREATMENTS

Chapter 10 The circulatory system   34

Chapter 11 The digestive system   46

Chapter 12 The muscular and skeletal systems   68

Chapter 13 The nervous system   80

Chapter 14 The respiratory system   94

Chapter 15 The skin   113

Chapter 16 The urinary and reproductive systems   135

PART THREE: IMPROVING YOUR VITALITY

Chapter 17 Maintain good energy levels   151

Chapter 18 Increase your mental and physical stamina   155

Chapter 19 Revive your libido   158

Chapter 20 Feel motivated and happy   160

Chapter 21 Defy the ageing process   162

Chapter 22 Make a full recovery from a serious illness   164

PART FOUR: CREATING YOUR OWN HOME APOTHECARY

Chapter 23 Buying from reputable sources   167

Chapter 24 Growing your own herbs   169

Chapter 25 Drying herbs   173

Chapter 26 Making your own tinctures, infused oils, syrups and ointments   175

PART FIVE: HERBAL FIRST-AID KIT FOR TRAVELLING

Chapter 27 Travelling in Western countries   181

Chapter 28 Travelling in remote and exotic places   183

Appendix 1 List of common and Latin herb names   185

Appendix 2 Glossary of actions   189

References   191
Bibliography   193
Resources   195
Index   197

Acknowledgements

I would like to thank all my patients who have given me feedback about their treatment; Katie, my best young patient who took herbal medicine although it was 'yuck'; all my teachers of herbal medicine who inspired me for life; my herbalist colleagues for sharing their experience; my family for being willing to try my unusual cures; my mother for introducing herbs into my life; my father for instilling a dose of healthy scepticism in me towards science and non-science alike; Neil Clarke LRPS for the photographic input; Monica French for her stylistic advice; my editor Amanda Cuthbert for the meticulous improvements to the book; Stephen Prior for his brilliant design; Alethea Doran, my copy-editor, for her amazing attention to detail; and the whole team at Green Books for their contributions to the final product.

To Richard

Introduction

This book is a simple guide to self-medicating with medicinal herbs. It deals with non-emergency first-aid situations and everyday ailments that people commonly treat with over-the-counter medicines. It focuses exclusively on using herbs as medicines and it is based on first-hand experience. All the advice you will find in this book has been tested in practice on my family, friends and patients. The main purpose of this book, therefore, is to share the practical knowledge that I have accumulated over the last eighteen years.

My confidence in using herbs for self-treatment stems not only from my experience as a herbalist – I was lucky enough to be brought up by a mother who was very knowledgeable about herbs and knew many home prescriptions for treating a variety of common problems. I have vivid memories of taking her remedies as a child: bitter chamomile infusion for tummy ache; tasty comfrey syrup for coughs; alder leaf plaster to heal a cut on a finger. These simple remedies worked every time, and as I grew older I acquired a deep respect for the healing powers of plants.

Herbs are the most natural form of medicine. Our bodies evolved to digest plants well and absorb all the nutrients. It follows that herbal remedies, being of plant origin, are easy for our digestive system to break down and assimilate. In fact, many food items used in appropriate amounts, for example garlic or thyme, become effective medicine. Unlike modern pharmaceuticals, which are normally composed of a single synthetic chemical, herbs contain hundreds of individual compounds. Herbalists believe that this biochemical complexity of plants matches the complexity of our bodies, and that is one of the reasons why whole-plant preparations can work very well in comparatively low dosages.

For centuries herbal medicine has been based on long-established patterns of use derived from empirical observations. Nowadays there is also plenty of scientific research to back up traditional use, and you will find useful references at the end of this book.

There are many advantages to being able to medicate with herbs: you avoid the potential side effects of many common pharmaceuticals (for instance, many people are allergic to Paracetamol), herbs are cheap and easily available (you would be surprised how much medicinal potential there is in the average spice rack), but most of all you will be helping your body to heal itself in a safe, natural way and not just suppressing symptoms.

At home I regularly use five medicinal herbs as teas, two types of skin ointments, about three to four essential oils and three to four specific blends made up from a few other tinctures. That is all. I do not need a full-blown apothecary to treat the majority of common health problems, and neither will you. The beauty of medicinal plants is that they are incredibly versatile: the same herb can be used for a very diverse range of problems. Take common chamomile: nausea during pregnancy, infant colic, indigestion, toothache, puffy eyes and acne are just a few cases where it could possibly be used. I have relied on my herbal first-aid kit on holidays in Britain and Europe as well as in the remote areas of Bhutan and Mongolia, and it fitted into a small plastic box. This book will help you to assemble your own individual herbal medicine chest to use at home, and a small first-aid kit to use when away.

All the remedies recommended in this book have been used by me and my immediate family on many occasions, and I do not advocate anything that I have not tried first hand. The treatment options that follow are all based on my personal experience, and have proved positive and successful over and over again. As a result, this book offers you a well-tested selection of effective remedies that will be appropriate for most families. I make it clear when you should seek specialist advice, as some conditions, such as eczema, although very common, are quite complex and tricky to treat by yourself.

The book is structured by the various systems of the body and their associated ailments, and my advice focuses on a few select herbs that can be used for several different systems. You will come across the same herbs in many chapters, but in each case a different set of actions and uses is described, relevant to that particular system.

This book aims to give you confidence in using herbs in preference to conventional over-the-counter drugs. If you are a health-conscious person, concerned with the quality of the food you eat and the impact of the environment on your family's health, this simple guide is for you: it will show you how to add another healthy option to your lifestyle – the option of natural medicine.

Part One
Opting for herbs

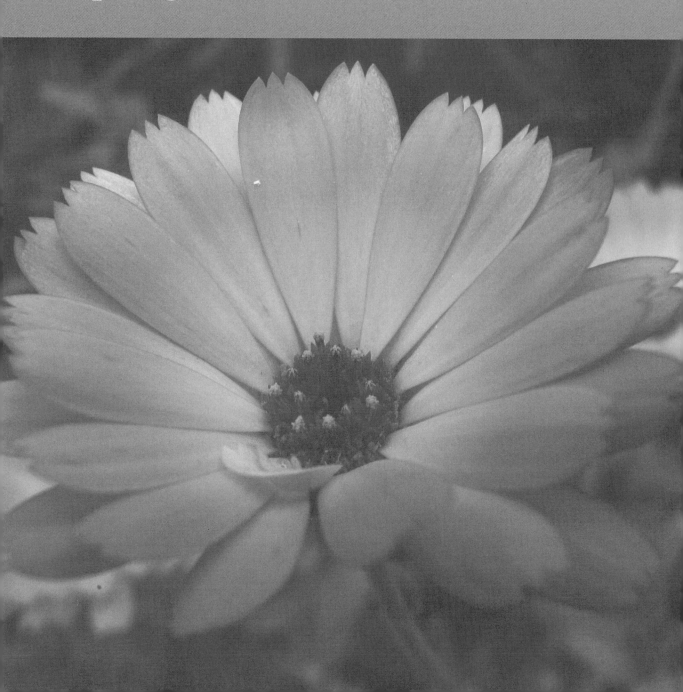

Chapter 1
Why herbs?

Herbs have been used as medicines around the world for millennia: they were the original medicine in all cultures and major civilisations. It is sad that, in many Western countries, the twentieth century saw herbal medicine being degraded to a complementary or alternative therapy, for it deserves a place in mainstream health care. Indeed Eastern countries, such as China, recognise the value of traditional medicine and incorporate it into their health care alongside their orthodox medicine.

So why should we go back to using herbs medicinally?

EFFECTIVENESS

In many instances herbs are as effective as, and sometimes more effective than, conventional pharmaceuticals in treating many common health problems. Did you know, for instance, that clinical trials[1] have shown St John's wort to be more effective than SSRI drugs in treating mild to moderate depression? Medicinal plants can often treat problems that defy modern medicine, including the common cold and chronic fatigue syndrome. They are equally applicable for ailments that arise suddenly, for instance heartburn, and for long-standing conditions, such as joint pain.

EVIDENCE BASE

The effectiveness of herbal treatment is backed up by many clinical trials. Therefore herbal medicine is an evidence-based treatment according to modern scientific standards.

Personally, I believe that the records we have of traditional use constitute valid evidence as well: our ancestors were quite skilled at treating everyday illnesses with herbs, even though they did not understand the nature of the disease. Today, we have the enormous advantage of being able to use the best of both worlds and combine modern understanding of what causes a particular ailment with traditional insight into which herbs best treat that ailment. A good example of this is the elderflower, which has been used for centuries by country folk in Britain and Austria alike to treat the common cold, but only relatively recently has it been shown to exhibit antiviral properties.[2] See the References for details of clinical trials.

LOW RISK OF SIDE EFFECTS

The majority of herbs carry an extremely low risk of side effects when compared with pharmaceuticals. But, although all plant medicines are natural, it would be naive to assume that they are all equally safe – some should be taken only with the guidance of a qualified medical herbalist. You must treat herbs with respect as you would any medicine: stick to the recommended dosage and make sure your information comes from suitably qualified professionals.

The herbs that I recommend in this book have an exceptionally good safety record and, as long as you follow the guidance for usage and pay attention to the cautionary advice, you are unlikely to experience any serious problems. Many herbs carry warnings, which normally means that they are not suitable for a very small proportion of people. For instance, in my practice I have come across one person allergic to echinacea and one to chamomile, yet these herbs are commonly used by a lot of people every day.

Some people may be allergic to certain herbs, and that is no different from being allergic to certain foods or to conventional medicines, and on very rare occasions some may experience a headache or a digestive upset. It is important to buy from reputable suppliers and rely as far as possible on native herbs to be safe, as some imported rare herbs have been known to be adulterated with potentially harmful species.

I would like to point out that the low risk of side effects applies to herbal products that have undergone minimal processing. Dry herbs and ordinary-strength tinctures are in that category. **Highly concentrated products, for instance essential oils, are not safe to be used internally and should be reserved only for external treatment.** All highly concentrated herbal extracts, which well exceed the concentrations traditionally used in the past, should be treated with circumspection. See Chapter 6 for more on the safety of specific preparations.

HELPING THE BODY TO HEAL ITSELF

Herbs help the body to heal itself, rather than just suppressing the symptoms. A classic example is the treatment of high blood pressure. The appropriate herbal treatment can not only bring blood pressure down but will also restore the healthy function of the circulatory system, so that after a period of treatment your blood pressure should remain normal without any medication. Similarly, taking echinacea will improve the function of your immune system, which will then be better at fighting off disease.

COMPLEX MEDICINE FOR COMPLEX BODIES

Medicinal herbs are complex mixtures of many constituents, which mirror the complexity of our bodies. Many of these constituents improve the function of a specific organ or bodily system so that the body can fight the disease more effectively. Herbs can harness our natural ability to heal: working along with our immune system, they gently nudge our bodies towards recovery. The constituents of herbs also have high bioavailability, which means that we absorb them well and therefore do not need large doses. Our bodies are adapted to digesting and absorbing plants, while many constituents of herbs are similar to those of fruit and vegetables and equally beneficial for our health.

Plants that are used medicinally can be viewed as a category of healing substances that sit somewhere between pharmaceuticals and food. Many have proven medicinal properties but are akin to food in their biochemical composition and the way in which they are absorbed. Some herbs are very familiar in the kitchen: garlic, thyme or blueberries, for example. Most are strictly medicinal yet gentle enough to be taken every day. Modern living has meant that people have grown so detached from nature that they can sometimes perceive the most natural medicine in the world as alien and hazardous.

The complexity of the biochemical composition of each herb is crucial to its effectiveness and safety. It is a modern misconception favoured by many scientists that a single substance makes better medicine than a complex mixture. It is easier to research, but is it better for our health?

Medicinal herbs are often referred to as crude medicines, and attempts are continually made to isolate the individual components to try to convert these into pharmaceuticals. Many medicinal plants have yielded or inspired useful drugs such as ephedrine, digoxin or aspirin. But considering the huge number of medicinal plants that are known, the quantity of single-component pharmaceuticals that have been derived from plants is relatively small. It seems that the active constituents of herbs rarely perform better in isolation. The reason is that plant constituents work in a synergistic way: the combined effect of many components is stronger than that of any individual component. Moreover, medicinal plants often display a curious combination of strong-acting constituents – which have potential side effects – with the protective constituents that moderate this potential. For instance, using dandelion leaf tea as a diuretic could lead to depleting potassium levels in the body if it wasn't for the fact that dandelion leaf contains enough potassium to compensate for the loss.

NON-ADDICTIVE

Another important point is that herbs that are used medicinally are non-addictive: you can stop using them at any time without risking the onset of withdrawal symptoms. This is especially important for people who suffer from anxiety, depression and insomnia, as they often become dependent on conventional medication. Most herbs can also be used alongside orthodox medication, although this is best done under the supervision of a trained medical herbalist.

AFFORDABLE

Herbs have the advantage of being cheap and easily available – you can grow some in your garden or in plant pots for your domestic use. Growing your own medicine is immensely satisfying, as it gives you a real sense of self-reliance. Whether you decide to grow your own herbs or buy them over the counter, you will be taking a positive step towards maintaining optimal health. You will be choosing an effective, safe and natural option; an option, moreover, that has been tested over many previous generations.

HAVE WE LOST OUR INSTINCTS?

Humans are not unique in using plants as medicines. Many animals – monkeys, horses, birds, cats and dogs – self-medicate with plants. Chimps have been observed to use herbs both internally and externally to get rid of parasites, stomach ache and itchy skin; presumably they have an instinct that guides them to the right plant for a specific situation. People who live very close to nature – the Amazonian Indians, for instance – claim that the plants themselves 'tell' them which disease they are for. One could interpret this as instinct or very finely tuned senses which develop when living in a natural environment. It is unlikely that people in Western countries have even a tiny remnant of that instinct, but we can learn from the knowledge accumulated by our predecessors as well as from modern scientific research into plant properties.

SEEK HELP IF NECESSARY

Of course, there are limits to what herbs can treat and there are situations where self-medicating with herbs is not the best choice, and throughout the book I make it quite clear when it is advisable to seek professional help.

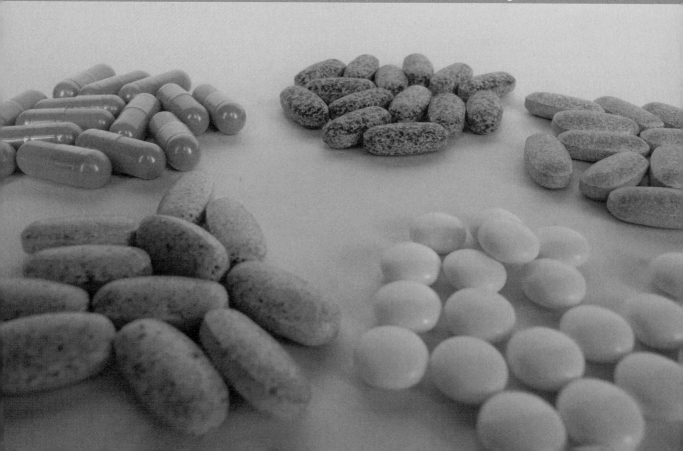

Herbal tablets (clockwise from top left): marshmallow root powder, willow, echinacea, garlic and milk thistle

Chapter 2

How to get the best from this book

This book is designed to be a quick reference source. If you have a particular health problem, look it up either in the index or in the appropriate section: for instance, if you have a cold, refer to the respiratory tract section; if you have stomach ache, refer to the digestive tract section.

PRECAUTIONS AND DOSAGE

Before you commence any treatment, I would strongly recommend that you read all the introductory chapters, paying special attention to the precautions and dosage chapters in Part One. The advice that follows in Part Two will make much more sense if you read these chapters, as you will become familiar with the terminology and concepts. This is particularly important if you have never used herbs as medicines before, but even a seasoned herb user should familiarise him- or herself with the dosage chapter.

IMPORTANT ENVIRONMENTAL CONSIDERATIONS

Chapter 4, on herbs and the environment, is also crucial – there are environmental reasons why it is preferable to use some herbs and not others, and if you want to be a responsible herb user this section is a must.

SUPPLIERS

Before buying any herbs, refer to the Resources section. It will tell you where to find a trust-worthy supplier, which is really important from the safety point of view and will also make a difference to your pocket.

IF YOU HAVE NEVER USED HERBS BEFORE

If you are a complete novice at using herbs for self-treatment I would advise you stick to one herb at a time before you go on to mixing different herbs together. That way you will minimise the possibility of any allergic reaction, and you will learn to observe the effects of any individual herb on your body. A lot of treatment advice in this book is based on single herbs anyway. Once you are confident with using single herbs, read Chapter 8 on combining herbs and then you can start mixing and matching different herbs to suit your particular situation.

Chapter 3
General precautions

FOLLOW THE ADVICE ON DOSAGE

The herbs recommended for self-treatment in this book are extremely safe, but you must follow the guidelines on dosage as strictly as you would with conventional medicine. Do not take larger doses than recommended and make sure that you adjust the dose for children, pregnant women and people over 70. General dosage advice is given in Chapter 6; please familiarise yourself with this information. More specific advice is given when discussing particular treatments.

SPECIFIC PRECAUTIONS

Please pay attention to the specific precautions highlighted throughout the book, as some herbs are not suitable for pregnant or breastfeeding women, for example, or for young children or people taking conventional medication.

TREATING BABIES

With one or two exceptions, I do not recommend that you treat children below two years old without first consulting a medical herbalist. I also advise against using essential oils for babies, small children and pregnant women without first consulting a trained aromatherapist or herbalist.

SEEK HELP IF NECESSARY

There is no problem with self-diagnosis and self-treatment as long as you can recognise situations where you should seek professional help. Use your common sense – if someone appears to be very ill, do not delay seeing a health professional.

The following are some of the symptoms that require prompt attention from a doctor.

- Prolonged severe pain, including constant head pain (irrespective of whether the pain has resulted from injury or not).

- High fever of over 39°C/102°F (invest in a digital thermometer – they are easy to use and read).

- Prolonged vomiting and diarrhoea (especially in small children).

- Marked changes in normal behaviour (especially in small children and the elderly).

You should also seek professional medical help if:

- you are unsure of the treatment

- you are concerned about any symptoms, even those that seem benign

- you are not getting better in spite of the treatment: you should normally expect an improvement within a few hours to a few days, depending on the problem

- the condition is long-standing or a complex one with many symptoms.

DRUGS / HERBS INTERACTION

In rare cases certain herbs can interact with certain drugs, so if you are taking medication prescribed by your doctor or hospital you should check with a medical herbalist whether it is safe to take herbs. You can ask your GP too, but unless a doctor is trained in herbal medicine he or she is unlikely to know much about herbs. In most instances taking herbs alongside pharmaceuticals is safe, but it is best to double check. It is also important to tell medical staff that you are taking herbs if you are about to undergo an operation or medical investigation. To be on the safe side, stop taking any herbs a week beforehand. Throughout this book I alert you to possible drug interactions when talking about specific herbs.

POSSIBILITY OF ALLERGY

Very occasionally, herbs can cause allergic reactions. If you develop any rash, itchiness, headache or stomach upset while taking a particular herb, stop using it immediately. If you are prone to allergies, watch out for herbs belonging to the daisy family, known as *Compositae* (examples from this book include yarrow, chamomile and echinacea) and use them in very small amounts to begin with.

RULES FOR SAFE HERB USE

It is sensible to follow a few rules for maximum safety when using herbs:

- Make sure you have the right species – refer to the Latin and common name list at the end of this book. Anything that you buy over the counter must be labelled with the full Latin names of plants.

- Make sure you are using the right part of the herb – there is often a marked difference in the actions of different parts of the same plant. For instance, dandelion root stimulates the liver while dandelion leaves are primarily a diuretic.

- Make sure you buy from a reputable retailer and use reliable sources of information. See the Resources section for more details.

- Always follow the advice on dosage and check any contraindications.

Chapter 4
Herbs and the environment

If you want to use herbs without contributing to environmental damage, the rules are simple: try to use native species or species that can be cultivated in the UK, buy herbs grown locally and organically, grow your own, do not collect from the wild, and never buy any endangered species.

LOSS OF WILD PLANTS

It is very depressing for a committed herbalist like me to learn how many herbs have become endangered and rare through indiscriminate harvesting from the wild and loss of habitat. For example, in the UK we have lost the lady's slipper orchid and sundew from the herbal repertoire – both herbs only just surviving in a few isolated spots. Worldwide, Korean ginseng is thought to be close to extinction in the wild, as is *Echinacea angustifolia*; false unicorn and golden seal have become rare, while slippery elm has become an endangered species. The destruction has been driven by demand, and although all of the above are very useful herbs indeed, they can all be substituted with other herbs possessing similar properties that either occur naturally in Britain or can be easily cultivated.

LOCAL OR IMPORTED?

The fact is that our native flora provides enough options to treat most problems and there is rarely a true need to resort to exotic, imported plants. Also, quite a few foreign herbs can be successfully grown in this country and can even have better properties: for example, British-grown lavender has a higher concentration of volatile constituents than lavender grown in France, although this is a Mediterranean plant by origin. By limiting yourself to herbs that are cultivated in the UK you will also be reducing the carbon footprint associated with their transportation.

However, as always, there is another side to the story. Some herbs can be grown only in specific climatic conditions, and such cultivation, assuming that it is organic, provides a livelihood for many people in developing countries. Similarly, some herbs are difficult to cultivate and can be collected only from the wild, and, provided that such harvesting is sustainable, it is a useful source of income for local communities. Some environmentalists even argue that careful harvesting from the wild can lead to the protection of the environment as it is in the interest of harvesters to look after the habitats of specific plants so as not to destroy their source of income.

A number of herbal product manufacturers are highly ethical and actively pursue a policy of minimal environmental impact, either through encouraging organic cultivation or ensuring sustainable harvesting by indigenous communities.

Sometimes growing and drying herbs in hot countries and then transporting them to the UK is more energy efficient than cultivating such herbs locally, especially if they require hothouses.

You need to balance all these arguments carefully. In my view, a sensible compromise is to use native and locally produced herbs by preference and to resort to imported ones only rarely, when you cannot find a local suitable substitute. Please make sure that imported herbs come from sustainable sources or are grown organically.

I would generally avoid fads for foreign herbs that occasionally pop up out of the blue and claim to be a cure-all. Exotic does not equate with miraculous, and there is usually a perfectly adequate local equivalent of such a herb.

ONLY ORGANIC

It goes without saying that medicinal herbs for sale should be cultivated organically – or, even better, biodynamically. It is better for the environment, for the plants and for you. A healing plant that contains pesticide residue is a contradiction in terms and should not be used.

Similarly, if you decide to grow herbs yourself you should do so in a completely organic way. (See Chapter 24 for information on growing your own.) At this point it is worth mentioning that by growing herbs in your garden or allotment you will be greatly encouraging local wildlife. Wild herbs often flower in a less showy way than garden cultivars but are loved by bees and butterflies, while the seeds are popular with birds. Like wild flowers, herbs attract natural predators and discourage pests. As well as your health benefiting from using herbs, your garden will be healthier for growing them.

COLLECTING FROM THE WILD

Many herbs are collected from the wild worldwide. This practice, often called wild harvesting, is not indifferent to the environment. In many countries the wild native flora is under threat owing to its disappearing natural habitat. Therefore any collecting from the wild is best done in a regulated, sustainable way by professional, contracted collectors who know how, what and when to collect in order to have the minimal impact on the environment. At present there is very little of this kind of control in most of the world, although there are many initiatives in individual countries to protect medicinal plants from over-harvesting.

Collecting herbs from the wild used to be a common way of obtaining herbs in the UK. However, nowadays there are a number of ecological issues associated with such harvesting. As elsewhere in the world, many herbs in the UK have become scarce as a result of loss of habitat or over-harvesting. Some herbs grow in proximity to intensely farmed crops and will be accidentally sprayed with chemicals; some grow near busy roads and will accumulate the air pollutants there. Scarcity of herbs in the wild has a wide impact on ecosystems, especially on insects and birds.

So, should you collect from the wild at all? In my view, no. It is best to grow your own or to buy ready-dried or processed herbs from an ethical supplier. Unless you are absolutely sure that a particular plant is so abundant that what you take will make little difference, please do not collect from the wild. Wild habitats have become so fragile that even collecting seemingly common plants such as elderflower or nettle may be harmful to the local environment.

I suggest that you ask your local Wildlife Trust about the plants you wish to collect. If you are given the green light by them, collect a small amount, just for your own use, and do not destroy whole plants. Make sure you have identified the plant correctly: there is no room for mistakes as some poisonous plants can look similar to non-poisonous ones. For example, a common mistake is to confuse comfrey leaves with alkanet or foxglove, or take alkanet for borage.

CURRENTLY ENDANGERED HERBS

Below is a list of some commonly used medicinal plants whose current status is endangered or threatened. The list is likely to change in the future as there are continual efforts made to ensure the conservation of specific plants, and some plants are also beginning to be cultivated. There are many international agencies that monitor the status of medicinal plants in the wild, e.g. CITES (Convention on International Trade in Endangered Species of Wild Fauna and Flora), TRAFFIC (Wildlife Trade Monitoring Network), United Plant Savers, USDA (United States Department of Agriculture), WWF (Worldwide Fund for Nature) and Plant Life International. You may need to search the Internet for the most up-to-date situation reported by these organisations.

Please refrain from using the following plants, unless you are certain that they are cultivated products:

Arctostaphylos uva-ursi (bearberry)
Chamaelirium luteum (false unicorn)
Caulophyllum thalictroides (blue cohosh)
Cinchona calisaya (Jesuit's bark)
Echinacea pallida var. *angustifolia* (pale purple coneflower)
Hydrastis canadensis (golden seal)
Panax ginseng (wild Korean ginseng)
Ulmus fulva (slippery elm)
Uncaria tomentosa (cat's claw)

CHOOSE THE RIGHT SUPPLIER

If you care about the environment worldwide, buy only from suppliers who will not sell endangered species and set strict standards for sustainable wild harvesting. A list of such retailers can be found in the Resources section at the end of this book.

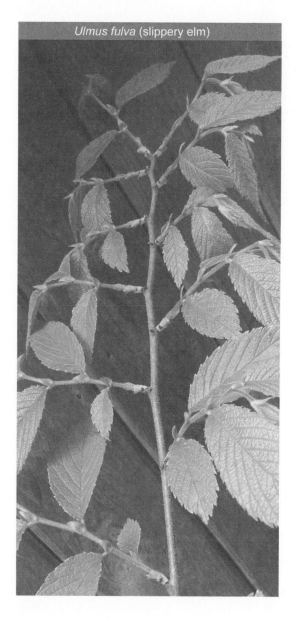
Ulmus fulva (slippery elm)

Chapter 5
Tea, tincture or tablets?

Herbal medicines come in many forms, and you may find some of them more convenient to use than others – or you may have a personal preference for a particular type of preparation. Throughout this book I usually recommend tinctures and teas (infusions) because they work quickly and you can easily mix two or more ingredients together, but there will be situations where a powdered herb or syrup is more suitable. Good-quality capsules or tablets can also work well, but make sure you buy them from a reputable supplier. You can take different forms of preparation together, for instance, garlic tablets and herbal tea. Tablets are best for travelling as there is no risk of spillage. The preparations most commonly used are described below, with an explanation of how to take them.

TINCTURE

A tincture is an extract that results from steeping herbs in alcohol for a period of time; during the steeping time active constituents from a plant dissolve into the alcohol. Specific proportions of herbs and alcohol are used to produce different tincture strengths or ratios. Typical proportions are 1:5, 1:3, 1:2 or 1:1, but occasionally you may come across different ratios, such as 1:8, 1:10 or 2:1.

To give you an example, a 1:5 ('one in five') tincture is made with one part of plant material and five parts of alcohol, both expressed in weight. If you buy a ready-made tincture the strength of alcohol used for making it will be indicated on the label, expressed in percentage, and can vary between 25% and 90%. It is important to realise that the term 'tincture strength' refers only to the concentration of plant constituents in a given tincture, and must not be confused with the strength of alcohol used for the extraction process. Tincture strength determines the dosage of a particular tincture, while the strength of alcohol is relevant to the process of extraction and the quality of the product.

CONCENTRATED AND STANDARDISED TINCTURES

I would avoid any tinctures that are highly concentrated (e.g. more than 2:1), as such tinctures have not been used traditionally and little is known about their safety. For the same reason I would also advise against using standardised tinctures, unless such a tincture is provided for you by a qualified medical herbalist for a specific reason. Standardised tinctures usually focus on one specific constituent of a particular herb and are guaranteed to contain a particular amount of such a constituent. In addition to the lack of traditional knowledge, there are also a number of other problems with these tinctures: they disregard the synergy between all the constituents of a given medicinal plant, they often choose a constituent that has been wrongly assumed to be the most active one, and they can contain an artificially high proportion of a particular compound.

DIFFERENT NAMES

You may come across different terms for tinctures: herbal extract, liquid extract, fluid extract or glycerite (based on glycerine instead of alcohol).

BENEFITS OF USING TINCTURES

Tinctures are easy to use, well absorbed and versatile in application. The amount of alcohol in each dose is negligible; therefore they can be used for all age groups, except for babies, and in pregnancy.

HOW TO TAKE TINCTURES

Warning: A dose of tincture must be mixed with water before drinking – do not take tinctures neat!

The amount of water used to dilute a dose of tincture can be as little as 30ml or as much as a full cup. It is a matter of personal preference: if you dilute with a small amount of water you have less to drink but the taste is strong; if you dilute with more water the taste is better but there is more to drink. Some people opt for the former and then follow it with a cup of plain water. Although water is preferable, you can also use fruit juice to dilute tinctures, especially for children.

If you want to make your own tinctures instead of buying ready-made ones, refer to Chapter 26.

INFUSION

Otherwise known as tea or tisane, an infusion is a hot-water extract of a particular herb or herb mix. I recommend that you brew a fresh infusion each time it is required. In theory you can keep an infusion for 24 hours in a fridge and gently reheat it when you need it, but freshly brewed herbs taste much better. You can use herbs available in tea bags, but for medicinal use brew them stronger than usual (two tea bags per cup). Infusions are the best way of administering herbal medicines for the digestive system.

TO MAKE AN INFUSION

1. Take 2 teaspoonsful of dry herbs, 2 herbal tea bags or 3-4 teaspoonsful of fresh herbs roughly chopped.
2. Put in an average tea mug or small teapot (you should be able to fill it with approximately 300ml of water).
3. Pour boiling water over the herbs, stir and cover with a lid or small saucer.
4. Leave to infuse for 10-15 minutes. Strain and drink while still warm.

DECOCTION

A decoction is also a hot-water extract of herbs but it requires 15 minutes of gentle boiling. This method is used for dried roots and barks. I generally recommend that you use tinctures of such herbs, but there may be some situations when alcoholic extracts are undesirable and you may need to resort to a decoction. You can make a greater quantity of decoction in one go by using multiples of the same proportions, and then keep the strained liquid for up to 48 hours in the fridge. Decoctions on the whole have a strong and bitter taste, and so are not for the fainthearted!

> **TO MAKE A DECOCTION**
> 1. Put 2 teaspoonsful of dry root or bark in a small saucepan.
> 2. Pour 1 ½ glasses of water over the herbs (about 400ml).
> 3. Bring to the boil and simmer uncovered for 15 minutes.

CAPSULES / TABLETS

These are very convenient to use. They usually contain either a finely powdered herb or freeze-dried extract. The quality is often an issue – use only well-known brands or purchase directly from a herbal practitioner.

POWDER

Powdered herbs can be taken mixed with water to create a protective coating for the digestive system. Powders of marshmallow root or liquorice are most commonly used, and they are great natural substitutes for over-the-counter antacids.

CREAMS / OINTMENTS

Creams and ointments are used mainly for skin conditions, and for muscle and joint aches. Herbalists make their own creams that combine base creams with tinctures, essential oils, infused oils, aromatic waters and infusions. Nowadays you can easily get hold of good-quality herbal creams, but if you want to make your own, refer to Chapter 26.

ESSENTIAL OILS

> **Warning:** Never use essential oils internally unless under the guidance of a health professional, as many essential oils can be harmful even in quite small quantities if ingested. Some essential oils are not suitable for pregnant women or babies.

Essential oils are highly concentrated products usually made by the steam distillation of plants rich in volatile substances, and they should not be equated with the plants they come from in terms of actions or safety. Essential oils come from plants with a strong scent, such as rosemary, peppermint, lavender, pine, etc. They should **always** be diluted in a carrier oil or in a cream/ointment for external application.

With one or two exceptions specifically mentioned in this book, I do not recommend using essential oils for children under the age of 3 or for pregnant women, unless under the guidance of a professional aromatherapist or medical herbalist. Many components of essential oils are absorbed through the skin, and if the dilution is too strong they can be potentially harmful, especially to babies or a developing foetus.

COMPRESSES

For a compress you can use cotton wool, a clean cloth or a flannel soaked in very warm (almost hot) herbal tea. I have found cotton wool the best, as it can hold more liquid without dripping than a cloth or flannel can. Place it against the painful area and keep re-soaking it every few minutes, as the compress works best when it is warm. If you want the compress to remain in place for longer, cover the cotton wool/cloth with a bit of plastic (any plastic bag will do) or Clingfilm, and then secure in the required position with an elastic bandage. The idea is to trap the heat as well as the moisture, so you should use a very warm infusion for that purpose, in fact as warm as you can bear, but be careful not to burn yourself.

Herbal tea bags (or ordinary black tea bags) can be used directly as eye compresses, but make sure that they are warm and not hot, as eyelids are very sensitive.

POULTICES

Poultices involve the direct contact of herbs with the skin. In my experience they work better than compresses, but are a bit messy. They can be made in two ways.

1. You can use herb powder mixed with hot water into a thick paste; put it on a clean cloth (lint or gauze) and apply directly to the skin, provided the skin is not broken. Marshmallow root powder can be used in this way to draw splinters out.

2. You can use fresh herbs, quickly scalded with hot water and drained, or dry herbs that are brewed to make a very strong tea (use twice the amount of herbs you would use for normal brewing, and infuse for 10 minutes). Squeeze the herbs lightly while still almost hot to get the excess liquid out, spread on to a clean cloth and apply to the sore area. It can be a little messy, but the direct contact between herbs and skin is extremely soothing and effective, especially for painful joints or muscles and swellings of various origins.

SYRUPS

These are strong herbal infusions mixed with sugar syrup or honey and used for coughs. You can buy ready-made herbal syrups from some stockists, but if you want to make your own, a generic recipe is provided in Chapter 26.

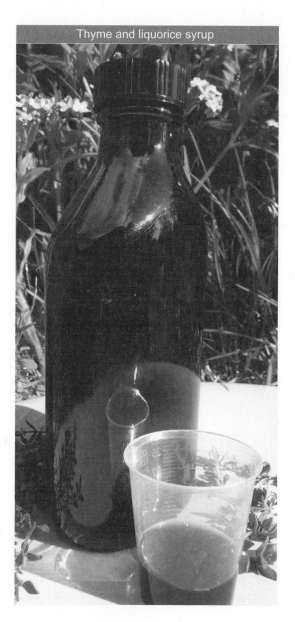
Thyme and liquorice syrup

Chapter 6
Dosage

Dosage is normally specific to a herb and its preparation, therefore you must follow the instructions from the manufacturer if you buy a ready-made product.

TINCTURES

It is essential that you understand that the recommended tincture dosages in this book refer to particular tincture strengths. Each dosage recommendation follows the same pattern throughout the book, for example: 1-5ml, 1-3 times a day, 1:2 tincture strength.

ADJUSTING THE DOSAGE TO THE SITUATION

As you can see from this example, a single dose can vary between a minimum (1ml in this case) and a maximum (5ml in this case). If you have mild symptoms you should use a minimum dose at the minimal frequency a day (usually just once), but if the symptoms are severe you should use the maximum dose 3 times a day. If you are of slight build you should opt for the small dosages, but if you are of large frame you will need dosages close to the maximum.

If you are not getting the desired effect with the minimum dose, increase it gradually, but do not take more than the recommended maximum. There is a large variation in what people need as individuals in terms of dosage, and it may take you some time to work out your optimal dose. Sometimes I recommend a specific dose for specific circumstances, which will differ from the usual dose range.

DEALING WITH DIFFERENT TINCTURE STRENGTHS

Because the dosage depends on the tincture strength and varies from herb to herb, it is not possible to give general guidance on the amount of tincture you should take. I suggest that you should try to obtain the exact tincture strengths advised in this book, which means that you can follow the advice on the dosage directly. If you have a different tincture strength from the one recommended in this book you must use the tincture according to the manufacturer's instructions.

MEASURING OUT THE DOSE

For practical purposes, 5ml is equivalent to an average teaspoon, but if you want to be exact you can buy measuring spoons or beakers from the chemist. Sometimes it is easier to use drops to measure out a dose. As 1ml of a tincture equals 10 drops, any dosage below 1ml can be easily converted to drops. For example, 0.4ml is equivalent to 4 drops. Use a glass dropper to measure out the drops.

TEAS

Herbal teas are not as concentrated as tinctures, so you do not need to be as precise with dosage. On average, an adult dose is: 1 cup of herbal tea, 1-3 times a day. This dosage refers to the method of brewing described on page 22. However, sometimes I recommend a strong infusion, which means that you add an extra teaspoonful or two to the normal amount and brew it for 5-10 minutes longer than usual. Conversely, if a weak infusion is recommended use 1 teaspoonful of herbs and brew for 2-3 minutes only.

ADJUSTING THE DOSAGE TO THE SITUATION

As with tinctures, the daily dosage depends on how severe your symptoms are. One cup a day constitutes a minimum dosage, and 3 cups a day is the usual maximum. Occasionally the maximum dosage goes up to 4-5 cups a day; where this is the case it is clearly indicated in the text.

ESSENTIAL OILS

Caution: I do not recommend using essential oils in external preparations for infants or children under 3 years old, or pregnant women, without first talking to a qualified aromatherapist or medical herbalist.

Essential oils should be used **only for external applications**. You can use almond, sunflower or hemp oil as carrier oils and dilute 5-20 drops of essential oil per 50ml of the carrier oil or 50g of the cream base. I generally recommend using essential oils in a bath, varying the amount according to age:

- children between 3 and 4 years old: 1 drop in a bath

- children between 5 and 6 years old: 1-2 drops in a bath

- children between 7 and 12 years old: 2-3 drops in a bath

- children between 13 and 16 years old: 3-4 drops in a bath

- adults: 5 drops in a bath.

Swish the water well to disperse the oil.

Please remember that many components of essential oils are absorbed through the skin, and if the dilution is too strong and too much is absorbed it can cause harm, especially to babies or a developing foetus.

ADJUSTING THE DOSAGE OF TINCTURES AND INFUSIONS FOR CHILDREN

Caution: I do not recommend giving a herbal preparation to an infant or child under 2 years old without first talking to a qualified medical herbalist.

In general, I advise against treating babies with herbs at home because babies need tiny doses and some herbs are not suitable. Having said that, a few common infant problems can be safely treated with herbs, and I give precise dosages for specific situations throughout this book.

You can use the following formula to calculate the tincture or infusion dose for children.

- Children between 2 and 3 years old should take ⅕ of an adult dose.

- Children between 4 and 7 years old should take ¼ of an adult dose.

- Children between 8 and 12 years old should take ⅓ of an adult dose.

- Children between 13 and 16 years old should take ½ of an adult dose.

- Children above 16 years old can take an adult dose.

If your child is small for his or her age, adjust the dose downwards. For instance, if your child is 8 years old but the size of an average 7-year-old, use the dosage for a 7-year-old. Do not adjust the dose upwards if your child is bigger than average.

PREGNANCY AND BREASTFEEDING

Caution is advised with many herbs in pregnancy, and some herbs should be completely avoided. If you are pregnant or breastfeeding please refrain from using essential oils for external applications without first consulting a specialist.

During pregnancy it is wise to avoid taking any medicines, including herbal ones.

However, some herbs are quite safe and can help with problems associated with pregnancy, like morning sickness. Again, I indicate clearly which herbs should not be taken while pregnant. The dosage for herbs that are safe in pregnancy may differ from the standard adult dose, so double check the recommendations for each herb.

Breastfeeding mothers can take the standard adult dose, but some herbs, e.g. sage and peppermint, should be avoided. This is because the active constituents of the herbs will be present in the mother's milk and ingested by the infant. Such herbs are clearly indicated throughout the text.

OLDER PEOPLE

People over 70 or those who are frail or of slight build should take less than the standard adult dose: $\frac{2}{3}$ of a standard adult dose or even $\frac{1}{2}$ if quite elderly and frail.

WHEN TO TAKE YOUR HERBS

Some herbs are best taken before meals; others afterwards. For example, to improve your liver function or increase your appetite you need to sip your (quite bitter) medicine at least 15 minutes before the meal, but if you experience heartburn you should take a soothing tea after the meal. Unless specifically advised, you should assume that the herbs should be taken before food.

HOW LONG TO TAKE YOUR HERBS FOR

An issue related to dosage is the length of time necessary to achieve the improvement in your condition. Most treatments recommended in this book are meant to be short-term: one or two doses to get rid of the stomach pain; two days of treatment to get rid of the cold; a few months' treatment to keep the hot flushes at bay. The general principle is that you take the herbal medicine until your symptoms disappear, and the longer you have had a problem, the longer it will take to get rid of it. If the period of taking a particular herb is crucial, specific information is given throughout the book.

If you are unsure about the dosage, or how long to take the herb for, contact your local medical herbalist.

Chapter 7

Choosing the right herbs for the situation

Choosing an optimal herb or herb selection for a given health problem experienced by a given person is quite an art. Not all stomach aches will be cured by meadowsweet, nor all colds by elderflower. If you don't match the appropriate herb(s) to the specific situation you will have poor results. Conversely, a good match of a herb to an illness will usually result in quick improvement.

Using herbs successfully is not a matter of using fixed prescriptions: you will need to learn to make individual choices for individual problems and individual people. It is not difficult – this book does not require you to learn about hundreds of herbs; on the contrary, I suggest that you rely on as few herbs as possible. But even faced with a small choice it is important that you select the best possible herb(s) for a given situation.

You need to take a number of criteria into account: the range of symptoms, their degree of severity, the age of the ill person, any other medication and/or supplements that he or she is taking, and so on.

SYMPTOMS

First of all, assess the symptoms carefully. For instance, if you have a cold, is it predominantly a runny nose, a sore throat or a cough? Or any combination of the three? Are you running a high temperature or are your muscles achy? If you have a stomach ache, is it related to something you have eaten or drunk recently, or is it a condition you get regularly when you

are stressed? Do you feel bloated or sick? Try to make sure you identify as many characteristics of your problem as possible. Decide which system of the body your ailment relates to and refer to the appropriate section of the book.

MATCHING THE TREATMENT TO YOUR AILMENT

Look up your illness and individual symptoms in the chapter you have chosen and familiarise yourself with the treatment options. Read the descriptions of the must-have herbs at the beginning of the chapter, as most treatments are based on just these.

Try to choose one herb that would treat the condition as a whole, but consider adding one or two more if specific symptoms are very pronounced.

Returning to the examples given above, elderflower would be good for a cold with just a runny nose, but for a cold with a bad cough you will need additional herbs, maybe a thyme and liquorice syrup. A cold with a very sore throat may require garlic or propolis as well as elderflower. Similarly, if you have a stomach ache resulting from possible food poisoning you may have to use garlic, charcoal and barberry, but if it is simply indigestion a meadowsweet tea will do the trick. The structure of the book will help you to get the right herbs for a given situation, and if you read the descriptions of individual herbs and indications for their most appropriate uses, deciding on the right treatment should not be difficult.

SPECIAL CONSIDERATIONS

If you are treating a child, see whether any of
the herbs are specifically recommended for
children and make these your first choice.
Also double check whether the herbs you have
chosen are suitable for pregnant women or
for people on conventional medication: if not,
look for alternatives among the optional herbs.
If you are already taking a herbal supplement
in the long term, do not include the same
herbs in your self-prescription.

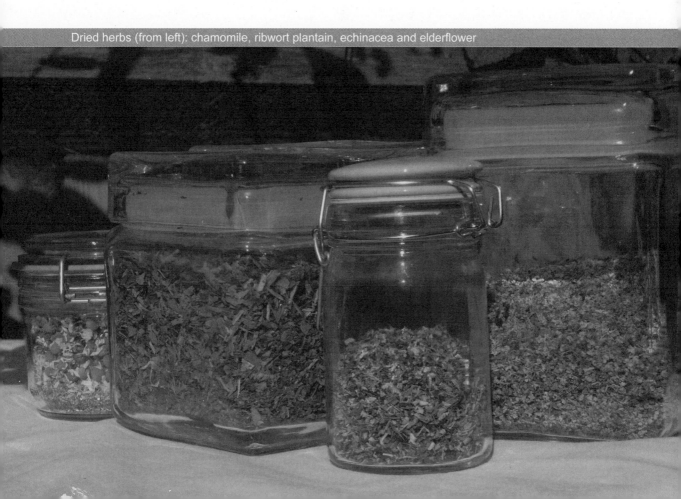

Dried herbs (from left): chamomile, ribwort plantain, echinacea and elderflower

Chapter 8
How to combine herbs

Some herbs go together better than others. I usually advise people to start using herbs individually, to get to know them well and then to proceed to combinations or mixes. But if you are feeling adventurous you may want to combine a few herbs straight away.

In general, you should combine herbs for their individual actions and for how well they work together. I have made suggestions for good combinations throughout the book, based on my experience. To begin with you can copy my prescriptions exactly to understand the principles behind mixing different herbs together. But in the longer term, following my suggestions for good combinations that are included in herb descriptions, you should try making your own herb mixes or combinations to match your individual needs.

COMBINING DIFFERENT FORMS OF HERBS

You can combine different herbs together as well as combining them in different forms. Tablets of one herb can be taken at the same time as a tea, tincture or syrup of another herb. Any combination of those is fine as long as you don't take too many herbs at any one time (stick to a maximum of five for any ailment). Some herbs work better in the form of a tea, others in the form of a tincture, so it makes sense to use the best form for each herb, even if using them together. You can drink herbal tea to swallow herbal capsules or tablets, you

can add tincture to the tea (not a great taste improver!) or you can take different forms of herbs at separate times if you wish. Throughout the book I suggest many useful combinations of different forms – you will notice that a tincture-and-tea combination is a common one, but if you favour tablets over tinctures, follow your preference.

RULES FOR HERB MIXING AND DOSAGE

There are a few basic rules to follow for successful herb mixing and for calculating the dosage of the mix.

• Keep it simple: stick to one herb for a particular problem to begin with.

• Add one herb at a time to your combination unless I specifically advise that more are included.

• Start by mixing the exact replicas of the herb combinations recommended in this book before trying your own.

• Don't mix herbs that do opposite things: for example, relaxing and stimulating herbs don't go together; neither do warming and cooling herbs.

• Two herbs with similar properties often combine successfully: for example, two relaxing herbs or two cough herbs will mix well.

- Try to put together herbs that will deal with different aspects of your particular problem, but use no more than five herbs at any particular time.

- When combining herbs in tincture form, use the minimum recommended dose of each individual herb.

- If you have combined several herbs into a single tincture, your dosage should be the arithmetical sum of the minimal dosage of each herb. For example, assuming that the minimal dose of herb one is 1ml, herb two is 3ml and herb three is 2ml, you should take 1ml + 3ml + 2ml = 6ml of the mixture.

- If you want to mix a larger amount, multiply the single dose by 3 to get a daily dose, and then multiply this by the amount of days you will need the mix for. So, taking the example above, let us assume that you want a week's worth of the mix: you will therefore need 21ml of herb one (1ml × 3 × 7), 63ml of herb two (3ml × 3 × 7) and 42ml of herb three (2ml × 3 × 7); and your dose will remain 6ml, 3 times a day.

- Always label the mixed tinctures with the ingredients and the date – you can keep the multiple compound tincture for up to a year.

- When combining teas, use roughly the same amount in weight of each herb and then brew the blend in the same manner as for a single herb.

- The dosage for herbal tea that is made up from a few herbs is similar to that for a single herb tea, i.e. 1-3 cups a day for an adult.

- Do not make more than 50-100g of a dry herb mix, as dry herbs do not keep as well as a tincture mix; make sure you label and date the mixture and keep it for no longer than 6 months.

Echinacea tincture

Chapter 9
What if it doesn't work?

You may sometimes find that the herbs you have used to treat a particular health issue do not produce the desired effect. Don't be discouraged, but look carefully at what may have been the problem.

- Your choice of herb(s) may have not been right for this particular illness. For example, if you treated a bacterial throat infection with antiviral herbs, you would not have much success.

- The herbs you used may have been of poor quality: this is an important issue, so please refer to the Resources section for suppliers of the best-quality herbs.

- You may have purchased the wrong herb or wrong part of a herb: double check the Latin name and the herb part (see Appendix 1).

- The dose you have used may have been inappropriate: refer to Chapter 6 on dosage.

- Your self-diagnosis may have been wrong: maybe you need to read up again on the distinguishing features of different diseases, or see a health professional to have your diagnosis confirmed.

Successful treatment with herbs requires some experimenting. We are all different genetically and we all vary in our response to herbs. Certain people will need larger doses than others and certain people will react well to a particular herb that does not do much for others. If you tried a particular herb selection from the must-have herbs and this did not sort out the problem, try some herbs from the 'optional herbs' selection, as they may suit you better. Observe your reaction to a particular herb carefully: for most conditions described in this book I would expect results from within a few hours to up to a few days. Once you have found a reliable herb that works for you in a particular situation, stick to it.

One of the reasons why I encourage people to try herbs singly to begin with is to see whether a particular herb does have a positive effect on the individual's body in the context of a particular disease. If you experiment with a lot of herbs at any one time you may not see the wood for the trees. Remember that the herbs recommended in this book are exceptionally safe: you are very unlikely to encounter any problems while trying out different options with them. The more you use herbs, the easier it will become to see whether a particular herb suits your particular body type, and you will start getting consistently good results.

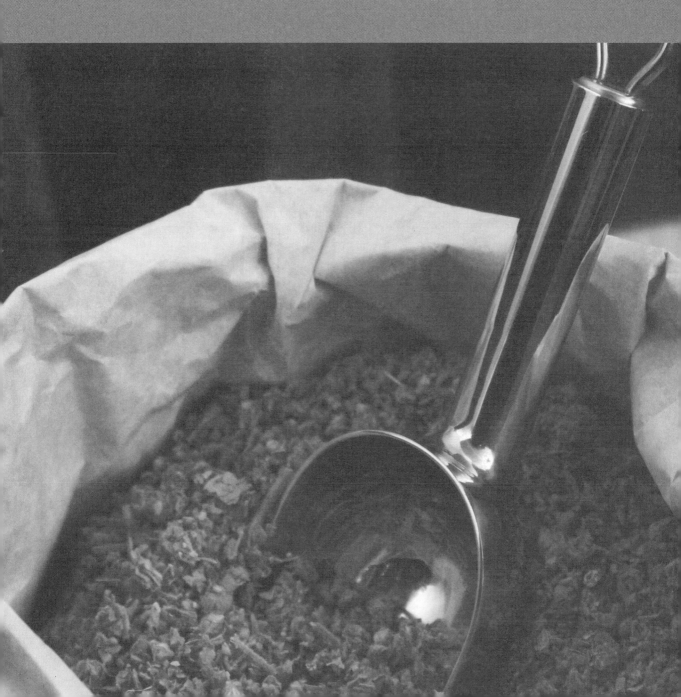

Part Two
Ailments and treatments

Chapter 10
The circulatory system

The circulatory system comprises the heart and all the blood vessels in your body: arteries, veins and small capillaries. Blood is of course a vital part of the system!

Disorders affecting circulation are very common. Mild problems such as chilblains can be easily treated at home, but potentially serious problems such as irregular heart beat require professional help.

WHEN TO SEEK HELP

If you are already taking medication prescribed by your doctor for a heart or circulation problem, I would not recommend that you try out any herbal remedies yourself. However, a medical herbalist may be able to advise you on remedies that can work alongside orthodox medication. Many cases of mild heart disease can be successfully treated by herbal medicine, but this needs to be done under the supervision of a herbalist, especially given that some of the more potent herbs are not available over the counter.

LOOKING AFTER YOUR HEART

Diet and lifestyle have a huge effect on the health of the circulatory system, which thrives on exercise and plenty of fresh fruit and vegetables, and which suffers badly if you smoke, take no exercise or eat too much junk food.

People are often confused about what constitutes a healthy diet for the heart and circulatory system, and many myths are perpetuated about what causes high cholesterol, which fats are good for you and how much red wine it is acceptable to drink. I strongly suggest that if there is history of heart disease in your family or you have been diagnosed with a circulatory disease you should see a dietary or herbal practitioner, who will be able to advise you on specific dietary requirements.

MUST-HAVE HERBS

The herbs in this section are arranged in order of usefulness.

YARROW

> **Warning:** Do not take if pregnant.
> **Caution needed** if allergic to the plants of the *Compositae* family.

Uses
Yarrow is a herb with many medicinal actions, one of the more significant being the ability to improve blood circulation. It can be used in many conditions where circulation is a problem: cold hands and feet, general sensitivity to cold, getting chilblains, nosebleeds, easy bruising, varicose veins or bleeding haemor-rhoids. Yarrow improves the blood flow to body extremities and reduces the tendency to excessive bleeding (hence its use in cases of

period disorders). It can be used directly on cuts to staunch bleeding. It is also helpful in reducing mildly elevated blood pressure, although it is best to have an individual dosage determined by a herbalist who can check your blood pressure on a regular basis.

Combinations
Yarrow combines well with hawthorn.

How to take
Either as tincture or as a tea.

Dosage
Adults: 2-4ml, 1-3 times a day, tincture strength 1:5; or 1 cup of tea 1-3 times a day.
Children (2-16 years old): adjust the adult dose downwards, depending on the age of the child – see Chapter 6.

GARLIC

Warning: Do not take large doses for prolonged periods of time, or when pregnant or breastfeeding.

Medicinal use of garlic is not recommended for children under 6.

Discontinue taking garlic 10 days before undergoing surgery.

Caution needed if taking anti-coagulant or anti-platelet medication.

Uses
Garlic is another herb that can be used for many health problems. It is a great improver of the circulation, and can prevent the development of clogged up arteries in people who are in a high-risk category (e.g. having a family history of heart disease, being overweight, smoking and having a high-calorie diet). It can help to bring high blood pressure down and keep your cholesterol low, and it also reduces blood clotting, so it can be very useful for people with a history of blood clots.

How to take
To be effective for problems of the circulatory system, garlic should be eaten raw or taken as tablets made from freeze-dried extract or freeze-dried powder (the effect of garlic oil on circulation is unclear). Raw garlic, finely chopped or crushed, can be added to food or each dose can be mixed with a spoonful of honey and swallowed. You may need to take large amounts for specific ailments, and if you are receiving other treatment it is best to talk to a health professional because garlic can interact with some medications.

To be of benefit to the circulatory system you should take only preparations that list the alliin or allicin content (the active constituents of garlic), and these should contain 5-12mg of alliin or allicin in a total daily dose. The tablets should also be enteric-coated to prevent the destruction of the active constituents in the stomach. Large doses of garlic taken for a long time can affect the digestion, so to avoid this take it for a month and then have a month off, or reduce the dose to the minimum.

Dosage
Adults: 1-3 fresh cloves a day; or 0.5-1g of dried powder in tablets (the equivalent of approximately 5g of fresh garlic); or 1 teaspoon of freshly squeezed juice a day.
Children (6-16 years old): adjust the adult dose downwards, depending on the age of the child – see Chapter 6.

GINKGO

Caution needed if taking anti-coagulant or anti-platelet medication.

Uses

Ginkgo increases the circulation to the extremities and specifically improves the blood supply to the brain. Although generally a very safe herb to take, treat it with respect: there are situations when it is best not to self-medicate with it – for instance, if you have high blood pressure, have a history of strokes or if you are taking blood-thinning medicines (you may still benefit from ginkgo but the dosage should be determined by a qualified herbalist).

If your health is generally good, ginkgo can be very useful to improve memory and concentration and also general blood circulation. It should be your first-choice herb if you always have cold hands and feet and do not cope well with cold weather. It is very useful when mountaineering in high altitude.

How to take

Tincture is the preferred way; make sure the tincture strength is 2:1 as the benefits from other strengths are unclear. Tea can be used instead.

Dosage

Adults: 1-1.3ml, 1-3 times a day, tincture strength 2:1; or 2-3g of dry leaf to make a cup of tisane, 1-3 times a day.
Children (2-16 years old): adjust the adult dose downwards, depending on the age of the child – see Chapter 6.

SPICES

Many spices, such as ginger, chillies, turmeric, cinnamon and horseradish, are beneficial for the circulatory system. They all have a mild stimulatory effect, which becomes obvious when eating any of these items – a feeling of warmth after having a hot curry is a direct result of more blood flowing through the capillaries!

OPTIONAL HERBS

BLUEBERRIES

Uses

Blueberries (and bilberries, which are the variety that stains the tongue and fingers black) are another example of food that is also a medicinal herb. Blueberries have an affinity to so-called microcirculation (the very smallest blood vessels in the body), especially at the back of the eye. Blueberries can help people who have sustained damage to the retina because of high blood pressure, and they generally restore the health of the blood vessels within the body. Eating blueberries will help in cases of virtually any disease of the circulatory system, and it will also have a preventative effect. You can eat them daily if you want, and frozen blueberries are as beneficial as fresh ones.

How to take

As food, either fresh berries or defrosted. You can also take a blueberry supplement in the form of tablets or capsules.

Dosage
Adults and children: 50-100g of berries a day. The supplement should be taken according to the manufacturer's instructions.

CHILLI (CAYENNE PEPPER)

Warning: Contraindicated with hiatus hernia, stomach or duodenal ulcer, and ulcerative bowel disease. Not suitable for small children.

Uses
Chilli peppers (Cayenne pepper) provide a great, quick boost to the circulation. They are best consumed as a food spice and can be included in your cooking on a regular basis, provided that your digestive system is in good shape. I would specifically recommend this herb if you get chilblains in winter and if you feel the cold easily (if you need to put on the central heating in September, eating chillies may save you a small fortune!). You can eat chillies in any form you like – powdered, cooked or pickled; food should be made moderately spicy to have an effect on circulation. If you develop heartburn you are eating too many chillies!

GINGER

Caution needed when breastfeeding, in cases of peptic ulceration or gallstones, and if taking warfarin. When pregnant, limit your intake to 2g/day of dried ginger.

Uses
This is a warming herb, which means that it improves the overall blood supply to all parts of your body, including the skin, hands and feet. If your circulation is not very good, particularly in winter, adding ginger to your food or drinking ginger tea will have a beneficial effect.

How to take
As a tea, made from fresh or dry rhizome, or use in cooking.

Dosage
Adults: 1g of fresh or dried rhizome 1-3 times a day as an infusion; or 1-3 cups a day if you use tea bags; or 1-3g of fresh or dry rhizome in cooking.
Children (2-16 years old): adjust the adult dose downwards, depending on the age of the child – see Chapter 6.

HAWTHORN

Warning: Not recommended for people with low blood pressure. Not always compatible with heart medication.

Uses
Hawthorn berries or flowering tops can be used to treat a wide range of problems associated with the circulatory system. This herb improves the function and health of the heart, it makes the peripheral blood supply to the hands and feet more plentiful, and it slightly lowers blood pressure. It can speed the recovery from a heart attack and stroke. It can be taken alongside orthodox medication under the supervision of a herbalist, but it is not always compatible with heart or high-blood-pressure drugs. For the purpose of self-prescribing I would recommend using it for poor circulation and slightly raised blood pressure.

Combinations
Hawthorn combines well with yarrow.

How to take
As tincture.

Dosage
Adults: 1-2ml, 1-3 times a day, tincture strength 1:2.
Children (2-16 years old): adjust the adult dose downwards, depending on the age of the child – see Chapter 6.

HORSE CHESTNUT

Warning: Do not take when pregnant.

Uses
The fruit of the horse chestnut tree is used medicinally to improve the health of the veins. It has a reputation for helping with varicose veins, but in my experience it mostly works as a preventative measure. However, people who suffer from varicose veins often have a poor blood flow from the legs to the heart, and horse chestnut will help to treat the resulting tendency to swelling. This herb is also useful for inflamed haemorrhoids and leg ulcers, as well as acne rosacea.

How to take
As tincture.

Dosage
Adults: 1-3ml, 1-3 times a day, tincture strength 1:5.
Children (2-16 years old): adjust the adult dose downwards, depending on the age of the child – see Chapter 6.

LIME TREE FLOWER

Uses
Lime tree flower, also known as linden, can help with raised blood pressure. It is suitable for people who are tense and stressed, as it is a gentle relaxant.

Combinations
Combines well with hawthorn.

How to take
Either as a tea made from dry flowers, or as tincture.

Dosage
Adults: 1 cup of tea, 1-3 times a day; or 4-10ml, 1-3 times a day, tincture strength 1:5.
Children (2-16 years old): adjust the adult dose downwards, depending on the age of the child – see Chapter 6.

ROSEMARY

Caution: Recommended only for external use.

Uses
Rosemary helps to enhance circulation to the muscles. The external application of preparations containing rosemary increases the local blood supply, and is felt as a pleasant warm sensation. It is useful for tired, overworked and achy muscles, which will recover much faster due to the locally increased circulation.

How to use
Rosemary is very useful as an essential oil, which can be used in baths or added to ointments.

Dosage

Adults: put 5 drops of essential oil in the bath and soak in it for 10-15 min. For an ointment, add 10 drops to 50g of the ointment base and apply to the affected areas 1-2 times a day.
Children (2-16 years old): adjust the adult dose downwards, depending on the age of the child – see Chapter 6.

VALERIAN

Uses

Valerian is primarily a relaxant for the nervous system, and as such it will help with disorders of the circulatory system that stem from stress, anxiety and tension. The range of problems includes raised pulse rate, heart palpitations caused by stress and mildly raised blood pressure.

Combinations

Valerian combines well with hawthorn and/or lime tree flower for the above problems.

How to take

As tincture.

Dosage

Adults: 0.3-1ml, 1-3 times a day, tincture strength 1:1.
Children (2-16 years old): adjust the adult dose downwards, depending on the age of the child – see Chapter 6.

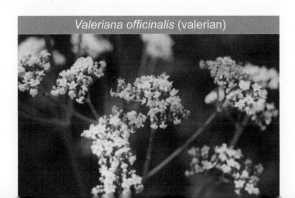
Valeriana officinalis (valerian)

SPECIFIC AILMENTS AFFECTING THE CIRCULATORY SYSTEM & HERBS THAT CAN HELP

ANAEMIA

> Practitioner treatment is recommended for this condition.

Anaemia means that your blood is deficient in haemoglobin, which carries oxygen in red blood cells. Usually anaemia results from blood loss due to injury, operation or excessive bleeding during periods. It can also happen as a result of your diet not providing enough iron or the iron not being absorbed from the ingested food. There may be other rarer causes of anaemia, and it is important to find out the underlying problem and treat it.

The main symptoms of anaemia are tiredness and shortness of breath on exertion, and many people do not realise they are anaemic until their symptoms become extreme. The measures below will provide good sources of easily absorbable iron that are free from the side effects associated with iron supplements. You could also eat black pudding, which is the best food source of all for iron, liver being the second best.

Treatment options

- Take an iron tonic, e.g. Floradix – this is a concentrated syrup made from yeast and herb and fruit extracts that are naturally high in iron (take it according to the manufacturer's instructions).

- Eat a variety of dried fruit daily (e.g. figs, apricots, prunes, raisins). *Adults:* a quarter of a cup a day.

- Drinking certain herbal teas will help, although this is not normally sufficient as herbs contain only small amounts of iron (useful herbs include nettles, couch grass, wild strawberry leaves).
  Adults: 1 cup of tea 2-3 times a day.

Children (2-16 years old): adjust the adult dose downwards, depending on the age of the child – see Chapter 6.

BLEEDING (CUTS, SMALL WOUNDS)

Here I am referring to domestic accidents such as cutting your finger with a knife while chopping vegetables (large cuts may need stitching), scraped knees or nipping your skin when shaving. The options below will help to arrest the bleeding, but if the cut is dirty you will need to clean and disinfect it, and then apply a suitable dressing if necessary. See page 125 for treating cuts and wounds.

Treatment options

- Use yarrow tincture diluted with cold water to reduce bleeding: either dab the cut or press gently on the area with cotton wool soaked in dilute yarrow tincture until the bleeding subsides (do not use neat tincture because it will sting). *Application for adults and children:* dilute 10ml of tincture in half a cup of clean water, as a one-off use which can be repeated if necessary.

- Use yarrow tea instead of the yarrow tincture (use either fresh or dry herbs). *Application for adults and children:* make a strong yarrow tea with 2 teaspoonsful of herbs per half a cup of water and use in the same way as diluted yarrow tincture.

- Use freshly squeezed yarrow juice instead of tea or tincture. *Application for adults and children:* juice fresh yarrow plants to get a few teaspoons of yarrow juice and use in the same way as diluted yarrow tincture.

BRUISING

Bruising happens when small blood vessels leak blood into the surrounding tissues. It is normal to develop a bruise after bumping into something or falling over. However, some people show bruising after minimal pressure to their skin and this indicates that the walls of their blood vessels are too fragile. The first measure given below is applicable to all types of bruising and is a first-aid item, while the other options deal with an excessive tendency to bruise and constitute long-term treatment.

Treatment options

- Use arnica ointment as soon as you have had an accident and you may prevent the bruise from forming altogether. Do not use on open wounds/cuts (although you can apply the ointment to the periphery of the cut, about 2.5cm away from the edge). *Application for adults and children:* apply generously only once on small bruises; larger bruises will benefit from 2-3 applications a few hours apart.

- Take a rutin supplement daily for a few months (take according to the manufacturer's instructions).

- Eat buckwheat or buckwheat flour on a regular basis (a good source of rutin).

- Eat 50-100g of blueberries a day for a few weeks, then reduce the frequency of eating to 2 or 3 times a week.

- Make sure you have plenty of vitamin C in your diet by eating at least 5 helpings of fresh fruit or vegetables daily.

CHILBLAINS

Chilblains appear on fingers or toes if you try to warm up very cold hands or feet too quickly, for instance in front of a fire or by getting into a very hot bath. They affect people whose circulation to the limbs is inadequate, resulting in very cold fingers and toes. Chilblains can be quite sore and red to begin with, and as they heal they can itch as well. If you are prone to chilblains you should take warming herbs on a daily basis through the winter months.

Treatment options

- Use calendula cream on chilblains as soon as you are aware of them. *Application for adults and children:* apply the cream generously twice a day.

- Take ginkgo tincture during the winter months (for precautions see page 36). *Adults:* 1-1.3ml diluted with some water, 2-3 times a day, tincture strength 2:1.

- Drink ginger tea regularly (for precautions see page 37). *Adults:* 1-2 cups a day.

- Incorporate chillies into your diet (for precautions see page 37).

Children (2-16 years old): adjust the adult dose downwards, depending on the age of the child – see Chapter 6.

HIGH BLOOD PRESSURE

Practitioner treatment is strongly recommended for this condition.

Raised blood pressure is a common problem which, if left untreated, may have serious implications for your health. There are many factors contributing to high blood pressure: diet, lifestyle, stress, genetic predisposition, level of exercise, etc., so it is important to address all the possible underlying causes. I do not advise treating high blood pressure at home, unless it is only slightly raised (135/85). If you do treat it at home you need to invest in a blood-pressure monitor to see if the treatment is working; if the results are not satisfactory consult your local herbalist for an individual prescription.

Herbal treatment of raised blood pressure is not normally lifelong. It will be long-term (6-24 months), but it often results in sustained improvement after that. The treatment options below should give you a cumulative 10-15% reduction in your readings (the optimal readings are 120/70 for a healthy young adult). Remember that blood pressure fluctuates all the time throughout the day and will go up markedly after drinking coffee or drinking alcohol (in the case of the latter the rise often occurs the next day).

Treatment options

- Take hawthorn tincture, made from either flowers or fruit (for precautions see page 37). *Adults:* 1-2 ml diluted with some water, 1-3 times a day, tincture strength 1:2.

- Take garlic, either fresh or freeze-dried powder in capsules (for precautions see page 35). *Adults:* 1-2 fresh cloves a day or the equivalent of 5g of the fresh plant in a dry form 1-2 times a day.

- Drink lime tree flower tea. *Adults:* 1-3 cups a day.

- Take yarrow tincture (for precautions see page 34). *Adults:* 2-4ml diluted with some water, 1-3 times a day, tincture strength 1:5.

- Take valerian tincture, particularly if you are under a lot of continuous stress. *Adults:* 0.3-1ml 1-3 times a day, tincture strength 1:1.

- Take the mix for raised blood pressure (see below). This mix should be taken instead of single herbs, not as well as. However, garlic is not included in the mix, so you can add it to your regime if you wish (for precautions see page 34).

Children (2-16 years old): adjust the adult dose downwards, depending on the age of the child – see Chapter 6.

MIX FOR RAISED BLOOD PRESSURE

Ingredients
- 30ml hawthorn (tincture strength 1:2)
- 20ml yarrow (tincture strength 1:5)
- 30ml lime tree flower (tincture strength 1:5)
- 20ml valerian (tincture strength 1:1)

To make
- Mix ingredients together.
- Pour into a clean, dark glass bottle.
- Label with the contents and the date.
- Store at room temperature for up to a year.

Adult dose: 5ml, diluted with some water, 2-3 times a day.

HIGH CHOLESTEROL

Practitioner treatment is strongly recommended for this condition.

High cholesterol is one of the contributory factors to atherosclerosis, which is the formation of fatty deposits in blood vessels. If these obstruct a blood vessel they can cause a heart attack or a stroke, so keeping the cholesterol at optimal levels is desirable. You can do a lot by having a sensible diet (eating no sugar and having the 'right' fats in your diet), and including lots of garlic in your cooking – or even better eating it raw. Having fresh, raw vegetables in a salad every day as well as a selection of fruit can lower your cholesterol too. If these measures are not enough, I recommend that you see a herbalist, who will advise you on specific herbs and supplements to keep your cholesterol down.

Treatment options

- Eat fresh garlic every day (see page 35 for more information about garlic preparations). For precautions see page 35. *Adults:* 1 clove a day, crushed and mixed with salad dressing or honey.

- Take garlic tablets (for precautions see page 35). *Adults:* the equivalent of 5g of the fresh plant in a dry form 1-2 times a day.

- Drink lime tree flower tea. *Adults:* 1-3 cups a day.

- Eat artichokes as often as you like, as this can lower your cholesterol level as well.

Children (2-16 years old): adjust the adult dose downwards, depending on the age of the child – see Chapter 6.

LOW BLOOD PRESSURE

Low blood pressure is normally not a problem. A small proportion of people with very low blood pressure may lack energy and feel cold easily. People who have low blood pressure should avoid any herbs that can lower it even further, e.g. hawthorn, yarrow or lime tree flower, but they will be fine with herbs that stimulate general circulation.

Treatment options

- Drink ginger tea (for precautions see page 37). *Adults:* 1-2 cups a day.

- Incorporate chillies into your diet (for precautions see page 37).

- Take ginkgo tincture (for precautions see page 36). *Adults:* 1-1.3ml diluted with some water, 1-3 times a day, tincture strength 2:1.

- Eat horseradish as a condiment on a regular basis.

- Take Korean ginseng as a tincture or capsules for up to a month (for precautions see page 153). *Adults:* 0.5-2.5ml, 1-2 times a day, tincture strength 1:2; or capsules taken according to the manufacturer's instructions.

Children (2-16 years old): adjust the adult dose downwards, depending on the age of the child – see Chapter 6.

NOSE BLEED

Frequent nose bleeds can be a sign of specific nutritional deficiencies, so if your diet is not perfect it may be worth seeing a specialist to get advice on improvements or specific supplements. However, sometimes it is due to a fragile blood vessel, or exposure to dry air or altitude. The measures below apply to people who have frequent nose bleeds, and need to know how to stop a nose bleed quickly as well as how to prevent it happening again.

Treatment options

- Apply yarrow tea to the nostril from which bleeding is taking place: soak a piece of cotton wool in the yarrow tea, squeeze the excess liquid, shape the cotton wool into a thin cylinder and push gently into the nostril, keep it there for a few minutes and replace with another piece if necessary.

- Drink yarrow tea for a month. For precautions see page 34. *Adults:* 1-2 cups a day.

- Take yarrow tincture for a month. For precautions see page 34. *Adults:* 2-4 ml diluted with some water, 2-3 times a day, tincture strength 1:5.

- Include blueberries in your diet on a regular basis for a while.

- Take a rutin supplement according to the manufacturer's instructions.

- Eat buckwheat or buckwheat flour on a regular basis (a good source of rutin).

Children (2-16 years old): adjust the adult dose downwards, depending on the age of the child – see Chapter 6.

POOR CIRCULATION

The signs of poor circulation are as follows: your hands and feet always feel cold or look blue in cold weather, you get chilblains easily or you find yourself dressed in twice as many clothes as everybody else around you! Energetic regular exercise improves circulation considerably, as does eating spicy food, especially chillies and ginger.

Treatment options

- Take ginkgo tincture (for precautions see page 36). *Adults:* 1-1.3ml diluted with some water, 1-3 times a day, tincture strength 2:1.

- Take yarrow tincture (for precautions see page 34). *Adults:* 2-4ml diluted with some water, 2-3 times a day, tincture strength 1:5.

- Take hawthorn tincture, made from either flower or fruit (for precautions see page 37). *Adults*: 1-2ml diluted with some water, 1-3 times a day, tincture strength 1:2.

Children (2-16 years old): adjust the adult dose downwards, depending on the age of the child – see Chapter 6.

VARICOSE VEINS / HAEMORRHOIDS

Practitioner treatment is recommended for this condition.

Although these two problems have quite different causes, they can both improve with a similar herbal treatment. If you are not getting satisfactory results with the measures outlined below, you may need more specific herbs that are best taken after consultation with a herbalist.

Treatment options

- Take yarrow tincture (for precautions see page 34). *Adults:* 2-4ml diluted with some water, 1-3 times a day, tincture strength 1:5.

- Drink yarrow tea for a while: 3-12 months if the problem is long-standing (for precautions see page 34). Adults: 1-2 cups a day.

- Apply witch hazel ointment to the affected areas 1-3 times a day.

Children (2-16 years old): adjust the adult dose downwards, depending on the age of the child – see Chapter 6.

WHEN AND WHY YOU SHOULD SEE A PROFESSIONAL MEDICAL HERBALIST

- Leg ulcers: these usually affect older people or those with diabetes; an integrated herbal treatment is needed, which comprises an individual mix for internal use to improve the blood supply to the leg area, and a special dressing to apply externally.

- High blood pressure: this is not suitable at all for home treatment as it requires regular monitoring and adjustment of the prescription depending on the results.

- Minor problems with your heart, e.g. palpitations and stable angina, respond very well to herbal treatment but they often require the use of herbs that are in the practitioner-only category.

- Very high cholesterol: you will need high doses of specific herbs, so this is best done under supervision.

- Frequent swelling of the legs/feet: this can indicate serious problems with circulation so it is best to see a health professional to establish the root cause of the problem.

- Acne rosacea: although affecting the skin, this is primarily a circulatory disorder. It is very difficult to treat yourself as it requires a careful adjustment of a herbal prescription.

THE FOLLOWING SYMPTOMS WARRANT SEEING A HEALTH PROFESSIONAL WITHOUT DELAY

- Severe chest pain, especially during exertion.

- Sudden, extremely painful headache and visual disturbances.

- Cellulitis: inflammation of the skin and small vessels, usually somewhere on a limb. Symptoms include: red, shiny skin, swelling, pain in the area and high temperature.

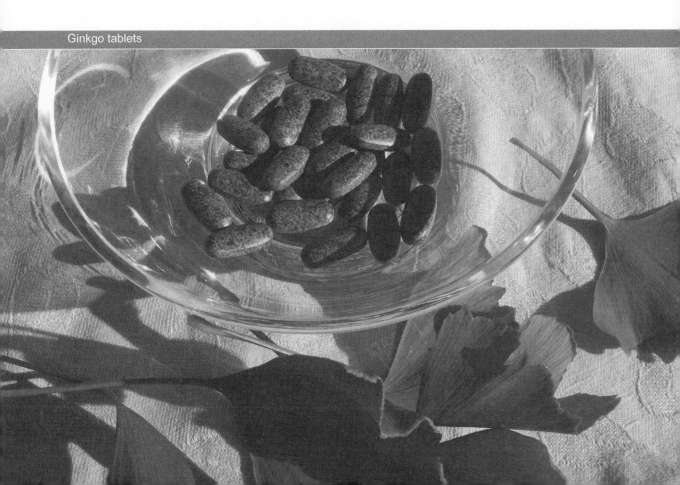

Ginkgo tablets

Chapter 11
The digestive system

The digestive system includes the mouth, oesophagus (gullet), stomach, small intestine (small bowel), large intestine (large bowel) and rectum. The liver and pancreas are two organs that are intimately connected to the digestive system and contribute vital secretions that enable proper digestion, but these organs are also involved in other functions. The liver is primary a detoxifier in the body and does many things: it stores quite a few nutrients, makes cholesterol, synthesises essential plasma proteins and removes worn-out red blood cells and some bacteria – to name just a few. The pancreas releases two important hormones into the bloodstream that regulate the glucose levels in your blood: insulin and glucagon. Most diseases of these two organs tend to be of a serious nature and I would advise you to seek professional help and not to attempt home treatment.

However, the rest of the digestive system is, in my experience, the easiest system to treat with herbs. The four herbs described below can treat most of the common stomach problems, such as ordinary indigestion, heartburn or bloating. They can be combined together or with other, more specific herbs. You can view these herbs as non-specific digestive aids – they bring almost immediate relief.

NUTRITION

Herbal treatment of the digestive system is more successful if combined with a temporary change to your usual way of eating. It is beyond the scope of this book to give detailed advice on different diets for different ailments, but the general principle in the case of any digestive problem is to eat easily digestible foods: plain white rice, simple vegetable soup, plain semolina cooked with water, plain couscous, weak black tea, steamed vegetables, poached fish or chicken. It is also advisable to avoid stimulants such as coffee, cola drinks, strong tea and alcohol. You need to maintain a plain diet only for short periods of time, sometimes a day or two, until your digestive function goes back to normal. Sometimes a day of fasting, with just water or diluted fruit juice, is a good option.

It goes without saying that a good, healthy diet is the foundation of the health of the digestive system and that an unhealthy diet will, sooner or later, cause digestive problems.

FRIENDLY BACTERIA

Many digestive problems stem from having the wrong balance of bacteria in the gut. This can be caused by having repeated courses of strong antibiotics, by ingesting unfamiliar bacteria when travelling abroad or by having an unhealthy diet. If you suspect that your bowel flora is not right, you can supplement your diet with probiotics, which is a collective name given to strands of friendly bacteria that normally inhabit the intestines, the most common being strands of Lactobacillus and Bifidobacterium.

USE HERBAL TEAS

The digestive system responds well to remedies that come into direct contact with its lining (mucous membrane). As the digestive system has a large surface area, it is logical to use remedies that come in large volumes in order to maximise such contact. Therefore teas are preferable to tinctures for stomach or bowel problems. **If you use a tincture for digestive ailments, dilute it with a full glass of lukewarm water.**

MUST-HAVE HERBS

The herbs in this section are arranged in order of usefulness.

MEADOWSWEET

Caution needed if allergic to salicylates. Seek professional advice if pregnant or breastfeeding.

Uses
Meadowsweet is extremely soothing for an irritated stomach or bowel, or any inflammation of the digestive tract. It can often relieve a digestive discomfort within minutes of drinking it. It is *the* tea to take after a late meal that is sitting too heavily, or to drink regularly if you suffer from reflux (heartburn), hiatus hernia or stomach over-acidity, and also if you are recovering from a stomach ulcer. It has antacid, astringent

and anti-inflammatory properties. It can be used for virtually any digestive problem, and I strongly recommend having it among your home remedies.

Combinations
Meadowsweet combines well with marshmallow leaf/root or with ribwort plantain, either as a dry herb or a tincture.

How to take
Meadowsweet is best taken as a tea and drunk after mealtimes. Brew fresh tea each time you need it and drink it warm. Fresh or dry herbs can be used. The tincture works almost as well as the tea, provided you dilute each dose with a full glass of warm water.

Dosage
Adults: 1 cup of tea 1-4 times a day; or 2-5ml, 1-3 times a day diluted with some water, tincture strength 1:5.
Children (2-16 years old): adjust the adult dose downwards, depending on the age of the child – see Chapter 6.

CHAMOMILE (GERMAN)

Caution needed if allergic to plants of the *Compositae* family.

Uses
German chamomile is normally sold under the name of 'chamomile' or 'camomile' in shops and supermarkets, usually as tea bags. Chamomile is an excellent herb to soothe painful conditions of the digestive tract, to reduce bloating and relax tension in the bowel. It is most useful for conditions

associated with anxiety and stress – so-called 'nervous indigestion'. Hence it is often helpful for sufferers of irritable bowel syndrome (IBS). Chamomile is great for children's tummy aches and for morning sickness in pregnant women.

Combinations
Chamomile combines well with peppermint, either as a dry herb or as a tincture.

How to take
Chamomile is best taken as an infusion. You can use either fresh or dry herbs to make the tea. If you decide to use tincture, each dose should be diluted with a full glass of warm water.

Dosage
Adults: 1 cup of infusion 2-3 times a day; or 3-10ml diluted with some water, 1-3 times a day, tincture strength 1:5.
Children (2-16 years old): adjust the adult dose downwards, depending on the age of the child – see Chapter 6.

PEPPERMINT

Warning: Peppermint essential oil should never be used internally.

Peppermint tea is not advised for children under 4 years.

Caution needed when breastfeeding.

Uses
This herb is stimulating to the digestive process as well as relaxing to the digestive tract. It will ease bloating and painful cramps caused by indigestion. Although peppermint helps to digest your food, it is easy to have too much of it, so in my view 2 cups of tea a day should be the limit. Peppermint tea can be too stimulating if you suffer from stomach over-acidity, hiatus hernia, reflux or heartburn, but it often helps people with IBS by relaxing the smooth muscles of the intestines. Peppermint also makes a refreshing and cooling drink on a hot day.

Combinations
It combines well with chamomile, either as a tea or a tincture.

How to take
Peppermint works best as an after-dinner tea, but it can be taken before meals to improve the appetite. I would recommend using fresh leaves if available (use 5-10 leaves, torn into smaller pieces, per cup). Tincture can be used instead of tea, but remember to dilute each dose with a glass of warm water.

Dosage
Adults: 1 cup of infusion 1-2 times a day; or 1-3ml, 1-3 times a day, tincture strength 1:5.
Children (4-16 years old): adjust the adult dose downwards, depending on the age of the child – see Chapter 6.

MARSHMALLOW ROOT POWDER

Caution: Marshmallow root can be taken with any conventional medication, but not at the same time: leave a ½-hour gap between the two.

Uses
Marshmallow root powder provides a protective coating for the lining of the gut as it releases its mucilage (slippery, gluey substance) when mixed with water. This

powder is a great option in any situation involving irritation or inflammation of the digestive tract, such as gastritis, heartburn, burning diarrhoea, diverticular disease, peptic ulcer, IBS, inflammatory bowel disease, etc. I use marshmallow root powder instead of the powder from slippery elm bark, because the latter is seriously threatened in the wild. If you are confident that your supplier uses a cultivated source, slippery elm bark can be used in all those situations where I recommend marshmallow root powder, in similar dosages.

How to take

You must always take marshmallow root powder with plenty of water (half a glass of water per teaspoon of powder). Mix a teaspoonful of the powder with some water, adding water gradually until the mixture reaches the consistency of runny custard, drink quickly and then drink a little more water to get rid of the taste. You can also mix a dose of powder with some yoghurt, which is a good way of giving it to children. Take this powder between meals for best effect.

Dosage

Adults: 1 teaspoon of powder, 1-4 times a day.
Children (2-16 years old): adjust the adult dose downwards, depending on the age of the child – see Chapter 6.

MARSHMALLOW LEAF

Uses

Use marshmallow leaves to make an infusion that will provide a gentle, protective coating to the digestive tract. Marshmallow leaves are similar in action to marshmallow root powder, but they contain less mucilage and are more pleasant to take. Like the root, the leaves treat many digestive complaints of an inflammatory nature, e.g. gastritis, heartburn, diverticulitis.

Combinations

Marshmallow leaves combine well with meadowsweet or chamomile as tea. I do not recommend the tincture for digestive purposes.

How to take

Marshmallow leaf should be taken as an infusion, either made with hot or cold water (see overleaf). Because it is a very light herb, use generously heaped teaspoons to make an infusion.

Dosage

Adults: 1 cup of hot or cold water infusion, 1-3 times a day (see box overleaf).
Children (2-16 years old): adjust the adult dose downwards, depending on the age of the child – see Chapter 6.

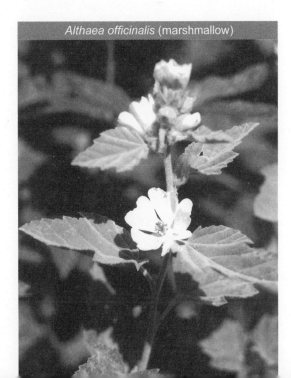
Althaea officinalis (marshmallow)

HOW TO MAKE A COLD-WATER INFUSION

Ingredients

- 2 teaspoonful of dry marshmallow leaf or 1 teaspoonful marshmallow root (not powder)
- 1 cupful of lukewarm water

To make

- Put dry marshmallow leaf or root in an average-sized cup.
- Pour a cupful of lukewarm water over the herbs.
- Leave to stand overnight (10-12 hours)
- Strain the herbs.
- Mix with some hot water so that you can drink it warm.

MEDICINAL CHARCOAL TABLETS

Warning: Do not take charcoal tablets or charcoal biscuits habitually for indigestion or flatulence because long-term use may be harmful – reserve them for emergencies.

Strictly speaking, this is not a herbal product, but charcoal does come from plants – it is burnt wood, after all!

Uses

Charcoal tablets provide a very effective treatment for mild food poisoning and diarrhoea related to eating suspect food. Charcoal works by binding to the bacterial toxins which cause the symptoms of food poisoning. This inactivates the toxins and reduces the symptoms while giving your body a chance to mount an immune response, which will get rid of the troublesome bacteria. Charcoal is not absorbed by the body but goes through unchanged, which means that it will stain the contents of your stomach black – do not be alarmed if you happen to be sick. Your stools will also become very dark for a while.

Combinations

Charcoal tablets can be combined with any other herbal treatment for food poisoning or diarrhoea.

How to take

You can either swallow whole tablets with water or herbal tea, or you can crush the tablets into powder, mix with some water and swallow the mixture. It is best to leave a short gap between taking the charcoal and herbs.

Dosage

Adults: Take 2 tablets with some water up to 4 times a day.

Children (2-16 years old): adjust the adult dose downwards, depending on the age of the child – see Chapter 6.

OPTIONAL HERBS

ANISEED

Caution needed if you suffer from reflux.

Uses

Aniseed is an excellent remedy for bloating and sluggish digestion. It is a gentle stimulant for the digestive system as well as a carminative, i.e. a herb that deals with excessive wind. It is a good alternative to peppermint.

How to take
The best way to use it is to add a few drops of aniseed tincture to water or any other herbal tea and drink it after a meal. You can chew a few aniseed seeds directly if you like the flavour, which is a common habit in some curry houses and greatly aids digestion.

Dosage
Adults: 1-2ml diluted with some water, 1-3 times a day, tincture strength 1:2.
Children (2-16 years old): adjust the adult dose downwards, depending on the age of the child – see Chapter 6.

BARBERRY

Warning: do not ingest when pregnant or breastfeeding.

Uses
Otherwise known as berberis, this herb is an effective antimicrobial agent for infections of the digestive tract. It can be used for gastritis, food poisoning, and diarrhoea of various origins.

Combinations
Barberry works well in combination with chamomile and witch hazel (see diarrhoea, page 58).

How to take
A tincture is preferable to a tea; take it either by itself or in combination with other herbs.

Dosage
Adults: 2-4ml diluted with some water, 1-3 times a day, tincture strength 1:10.
Children (2-16 years old): adjust the adult dose downwards, depending on the age of the child – see Chapter 6.

DANDELION ROOT

Caution needed if allergic to plants of the *Compositae* family.

Uses
Both dandelion root and leaves are used medicinally, but for digestive complaints the root is the part you need. Dandelion root stimulates the liver to produce more bile, which in turn means better digestion of fatty food. If you find that fatty food, such as bacon or full-fat cheese, makes you feel heavy and bloated, then taking dandelion will help. Of course, fatty food is not good for us and it is best to avoid it; nevertheless you should be able to digest such food without trouble; if you don't, then your liver may be a bit sluggish.

How to take
Dandelion root can be taken as an infusion, decoction (stronger in taste and action than an infusion), dandelion coffee or tincture. They all have a bitter taste.

Dosage
Adults: 1 cup of decoction 1-2 times a day; or 1 cup of infusion 1-2 times a day; or 1 cup of dandelion coffee 1-2 times a day; or 3-5ml diluted with water, 1-3 times a day, tincture strength 1:5.
Children (2-16 years old): adjust the adult dose

downwards, depending on the age of the child – see Chapter 6.

GARLIC

> **Warning:** Do not take large doses for prolonged periods of time or when pregnant or breastfeeding.
>
> Not suitable for children under 6.
>
> **Caution needed** if taking anti-coagulant or anti-platelet medication.

Uses
Garlic acts against a wide spectrum of bacteria that can cause digestive upsets. It can be used for mild food poisoning, traveller's diarrhoea, or as a preventative treatment when travelling in exotic countries. It can also be of help for some worm infestations (see page 66).

How to take
For the treatment of digestive problems you can take either fresh or processed garlic. Fresh garlic should be crushed or juiced, while processed garlic can be in the form of tincture, preserved juice, tablets or capsules.

Some people do not tolerate fresh garlic very well, so try a small amount if you have never taken it before. Young garlic is more likely to cause an adverse reaction. You can take garlic at the same time as demulcent (anti-irritant) herbs, such as marshmallow or linseed, to reduce the possibility of irritation.

Dosage
Adults: 0.5-1g of dry powder equivalent in tablets or capsules, 1-3 times a day; or 1 crushed clove, 1-3 times a day, with plenty of water; or 2-4ml diluted with water, 1-3 times a day, tincture strength 1:1; or 1 teaspoon of garlic juice diluted with water, 1-3 times a day. *Children (6-16 years old):* adjust the adult dose downwards, depending on the age of the child – see Chapter 6.

GINGER

> **Caution needed** when breastfeeding, in cases of peptic ulceration or gallstones, and if taking warfarin.
>
> When pregnant limit your intake to 2g/day of dried ginger.

Uses
Ginger is a warming herb that gently stimulates digestion. It also stops the feeling of nausea, including nausea during pregnancy, and car or sea sickness.

Combinations
If you suffer from reflux, ginger tea may be slightly irritating for the inflamed gullet, so mix it with marshmallow leaf; otherwise drink it by itself or with a slice of lemon.

How to take
It is best taken as a tea, made either with a slice of fresh ginger (1g) or a teaspoon of dry ginger powder (1g). Ginger tea bags are just fine.

Dosage
Adults: 1 cup of infusion 1-3 times a day. *Children (2-16 years old):* adjust the adult dose downwards, depending on the age of the child – see Chapter 6.

LEMON BALM

Uses
Lemon balm is a superb digestive tea that also makes you relaxed and ensures good sleep. When it starts growing fresh in my garden in the spring and summer, I often give it to my dinner guests at the end of the evening to aid their digestion, and many have commented how well they slept afterwards. Lemon balm infusion, made from fresh leaves, has a wonderful green colour, zesty scent and a fresh lemony taste. This tea, whether made from the fresh or the dry herb, is good for people whose digestive problems stem from anxiety, as it is both a digestive aid and a relaxant to the nervous system.

Combinations
It combines well with chamomile and/or meadowsweet, either fresh or dry.

How to take
Use a good handful of fresh leaves (not twigs), shredded into smaller pieces, per pint-sized teapot. You can add honey to this tea, or even a slice of lemon to enhance the natural taste. Dry lemon balm can be used for tea outside the growing season, but is nowhere near as tasty. It is very hard to get a good-quality lemon balm tincture, and tincture made from fresh herbs is preferable to one made from dry herbs.

Dosage
Adults: 1 cup of infusion 1-3 times a day; or 2-6ml diluted with some water, 1-3 times a day, tincture strength 1:5.
Children (2-16 years old): adjust the adult dose downwards, depending on the age of the child – see Chapter 6.

LINSEED

Uses
I recommend using linseed for the improvement of digestion in quite a range of situations. As a general rule, you can use it when bowel movements are not right, or when there is inflammation somewhere in the digestive tract. Examples of ailments that will be better for the daily use of linseed include: constipation, diarrhoea, diverticular disease, IBS, gastritis, and peptic ulcers.

How to take
If you want to get the full benefit of the linseed, you must **soak it** before use. The simplest way to do this is to put a tablespoon of linseed in a cup, fill it with lukewarm water and leave to stand overnight, stir it well in the morning and drink both the liquid and the seeds. Eating dry linseed (many people sprinkle linseed on their cereal or salad) will do virtually nothing, as the seeds will not have enough time to release the beneficial mucilage before they are excreted.

Dosage
Adults: 1-2 tablespoons of soaked seeds, once a day.
Children (2-16 years old): adjust the adult dose downwards, depending on the age of the child – see Chapter 6.

LIQUORICE

Warning: Do not take if you have high blood pressure, low potassium, heart/kidney/liver problems or water retention.

Caution needed when pregnant or if elderly.

Uses

Liquorice (or licorice) is a soother to the lining of the gut and therefore suitable for any condition that leads to the irritation of the intestinal lining. As such it is similar to marshmallow, but it also has a pronounced anti-inflammatory action. It is especially suitable for people who suffer from digestive problems owing to stress, provided that they do not have high blood pressure.

How to take

You can take liquorice either as tincture or as powder. The powder needs to be mixed with half a cup of water before swallowing. If you suffer from mildly raised blood pressure you can still use liquorice, but only in small doses and for short periods of time (half the normal dose for no longer than a week).

Dosage

Adults: 0.4-1.6ml diluted with some water, 1-3 times a day, tincture strength 1:1; or 1g of powder 1-3 times a day.
Children (2-16 years old): adjust the adult dose downwards, depending on the age of the child – see Chapter 6.

MILK THISTLE

Caution needed if allergic to plants of the *Compositae* family.

Uses

Milk thistle (St Mary's thistle) is a very specific herb: the seed extract protects the liver from the harmful effects of many toxic substances and also helps the liver to regenerate if it has been damaged by disease. Milk thistle

tincture is appropriate for a liver that needs support, but I recommend that you consult a herbalist before using this herb to make sure that you use it in the right capacity. The only situation in which I would advocate home use is after drinking a lot of alcohol – it will help you to recover from an occasional hangover (but it is not an excuse to drink more!).

How to take

Either as tincture or as powder.

Dosage

Adults: 1.3-2.6ml diluted with some water, 1-3 times a day, tincture strength 1:1; or 1.3-2.6g, 1-3 times a day of herb powder.
Children (2-16 years old): adjust the adult dose downwards, depending on the age of the child – see Chapter 6.

RASPBERRY LEAF

Warning: Not recommended in the first trimester of pregnancy.

Uses

Raspberry leaf is a gentle astringent for the digestive system and provides a very pleasant tea to deal with diarrhoea of various origins. Generally, it is not astringent enough to deal with diarrhoea caused by food poisoning, but is effective enough for a stomach bug (viral infection of the digestive tract), mild traveller's diarrhoea, children's diarrhoea, diarrhoea caused by antibiotics (in which case it is a good idea to take a probiotics supplement as well), some forms of IBS and even some cases of inflammatory bowel disease.

Combinations

It is best to mix raspberry leaf with meadowsweet and chamomile in equal quantities for the above purposes. You can use fresh or dry leaves, and, although wild raspberry leaves are preferable, any garden variety can be used as well.

How to take

As a tea, either by itself or in a combination with meadowsweet and chamomile.

Dosage

Adults: 1 cup of an infusion, 1-3 times a day.
Children (2-16 years old): adjust the adult dose downwards, depending on the age of the child – see Chapter 6.

VERVAIN

Uses

Vervain is for people whose digestion suffers when they feel low: it improves the digestive function at the same time as lifting the sufferer's spirit. It is useful for non-specific problems, such as in cases where your stomach or bowel just doesn't feel right but you can't identify any particular problem. For example, women can often experience digestive disturbances together with mood swings just before their period, and vervain tea is a suitable choice in this situation.

Similarly, people with chronic fatigue syndrome often complain about non-specific digestive problems; again, vervain tea will often help.

Combinations

Vervain combines well with chamomile and/or with peppermint, either as a tea or tincture.

How to take

Vervain makes a pleasant tea and can be drunk regularly every day by people whose digestion is easily effected by stress and anxiety, especially when their appetite diminishes. It is best to drink it in the evening in such cases. Tincture can be used instead of tea.

Dosage

Adults: 1 cup of infusion, 1-2 times a day; or 1-2ml diluted with some water, 1-3 times a day, tincture strength 1:2.
Children (2-16 years old): adjust the adult dose downwards, depending on the age of the child – see Chapter 6.

WITCH HAZEL LEAF

Uses

The primary use of witch hazel is for really bad diarrhoea resulting from eating or drinking something dubious. It is a very astringent herb and should therefore be reserved for extreme situations. Witch hazel is also used externally for haemorrhoids (see page 62).

Combinations

Witch hazel can be combined with an antimicrobial herb (barberry or garlic) and an anti-inflammatory herb (chamomile or liquorice) for the treatment of diarrhoea (see page 58 for details of mixing and dosage).

How to take

Witch hazel is best taken in tincture form.

Dosage

Adults: 1-2ml diluted with some water, 1-3 times a day, tincture strength 1:2.

Children (2-16 years old): adjust the adult dose downwards, depending on the age of the child – see Chapter 6.

SPECIFIC AILMENTS AFFECTING THE DIGESTIVE SYSTEM & HERBS THAT CAN HELP

APPETITE, LACK OF

Lack of appetite can be the result of an illness or poor liver function. Bitter herbs restore appetite and improve the general digestion. These herbs must be taken about 15-30 minutes before eating, and the bitter taste needs to be 'tasted', which means slow sipping rather than quick gulping. Many herbs have a bitter taste and the degree of bitterness often depends on how long a herb is steeped for when making a tisane.

For the purpose of stimulating appetite, tinctures work as well as teas provided that they taste bitter. If an illness is causing the appetite problem, try to treat that in the first place. If you are suffering from liver or gall-bladder disease, consult a herbalist before taking bitter herbs.

Treatment options

- Drink chamomile or vervain tea (for precautions see page 47). *Adults:* 1-2 cups a day, before meals.

- Take dandelion root tincture, diluted in half a cup of room-temperature water, and sip slowly before meals (for precautions see page 51). *Adults:* 3-5ml diluted with some water, 3 times a day, tincture strength 1:5.

- Drink dandelion root infusion (for precautions see page 51). *Adults:* 1-2 cups a day.

- Take barberry in a tincture form, diluted in half a cup of room-temperature water, and sip slowly before meals (for precautions see page 51). *Adults:* 2-4ml diluted with some water, 3 times a day, tincture strength 1:10.

- Add some warming herbs such as ginger or cinnamon powder to the bitter tea/tincture; put a pinch of either of the powders in the cup before brewing.

Children (2-16 years old): adjust the adult dose downwards, depending on the age of the child – see Chapter 6.

BLOATING

Bloating is a subjective feeling of fullness in your abdomen not necessarily related to the actual expansion of your waistline or the amount of gas produced. It usually indicates poor digestive function and a shortage of friendly bacteria in your bowels. Sometimes people suffer from sensitivities to common foods such as wheat, yeast or cow's milk, and you can try removing such products from your diet for a while. Modern bread seems to cause bloating in a lot of people: try yeast-free breads, based on sourdough. Some foods, such as cabbage, beans and lentils, are hard to digest for almost everybody – it is a good idea to add caraway seeds to these while cooking to aid the digestion. If you suffer from IBS, bloating will be one of the symptoms, and you will find that the herbs recommended below offer relief. However, as IBS is a complex condition you will get much better overall results from treatment designed specifically for your particular symptoms.

Treatment options

- Drink chamomile tea (for precautions see page 47). *Adults:* 1 cup after each meal.

- Drink peppermint tea (for precautions see page 48). *Adults :* 1 cup after lunch and 1 cup after dinner.

- Drink combined peppermint and chamomile tea (for precautions see pages 47 and 48). *Adults:* 1 cup after each meal.

- Supplement with probiotics for a month (follow the manufacturer's instructions); eating bio-yoghurts can be helpful as well.

Children (2-16 years old): adjust the adult dose downwards, depending on the age of the child – see Chapter 6.

COLIC (BABY COLIC)

Colic usually refers to baby colic – a painful condition that some babies are afflicted with. The treatment is delivered 'through' the mother's milk or added to formula milk. Use only tea – not a tincture – and don't brew it too strong (2-3 minutes).

Adults who experience a sudden colicky pain may be suffering from gallstones and must see a doctor. At times, both adults and children can experience colicky pain caused by trapped wind (see the treatment for excess wind, page 59).

Treatment options

- If you are breastfeeding, you can drink fennel tea, using one fennel tea bag per cup, and enough fennel will pass into the milk to get rid of your baby's colic – milk production may increase too! *Breastfeeding mothers*: 1-2 cups a day.

- Add a tiny amount of fennel **tea** to the baby's formula milk. *Babies:* 5-10 drops per bottle.

- You can use chamomile tea in a similar way to fennel tea.

CONSTIPATION

Constipation is an extremely common condition that may have many causes. It is often related to an unbalanced diet, lack of exercise and inadequate water intake. Soft fruit such as kiwis and plums will often sort it out, and you should also make sure you take in about 2 litres of liquid every day (include all drinks and soup, but not coffee or alcohol, in that total). The herbs listed below can be used in pregnancy, unlike strong herbal laxatives, which should not be used.

Treatment options

- Take linseed. *Adults:* 1-2 tablespoons of linseed. Soak in a cup of warm water overnight and drink both the liquid and the seeds in the morning.

- Take psyllium seeds. *Adults:* 1 teaspoon of seeds mixed with a glass of water once a day.

- Drink dandelion root tea: this herb stimulates the liver and improves overall digestion (for precautions see page 51). Adults: 1-2 cups a day; 1 cup if pregnant).

- Take yellow dock tincture, which has mild laxative properties; do not use this herb if breastfeeding, because it can cause diarrhoea in your baby.
  Adults: 1-2ml diluted with some water, 1-3 times a day, tincture strength 1:5.

Children (2-16 years old): adjust the adult dose downwards, depending on the age of the child – see Chapter 6.

DIARRHOEA

Diarrhoea is a symptom of many diseases. The recommendations for treatment included here refer to the simple, occasional looseness of stool that we all experience after a suspect meal or when eating unfamiliar food abroad. If your diarrhoea does not improve within 24 hours or is exceptionally watery you must seek medical help, as there is a danger of dehydration. This is especially important with small children, who can get dehydrated rapidly, so make sure that they drink a lot. Water with lemon juice and honey is good, or any diluted fruit juice.

Very strong black tea (no milk or sugar) can be helpful for diarrhoea if you have no access to other medication. Rehydrating powder available from the chemist (for instance Dioralyte) should be taken if your diarrhoea is severe and lasts longer than a day.

Treatment options

- Take a specific 'anti-diarrhoea mix' – see box, right. This mix has proved itself very effective on a number of occasions when I was travelling in Asia.

- It is good to take charcoal tablets as well as the above tincture mix, as charcoal absorbs toxins produced by the bacteria that cause diarrhoea. It is better to take the tincture first, and follow with the charcoal about 10-15 minutes later, otherwise the charcoal may inactivate some of the herbal constituents of the tincture. *Adults:* 2 tablets up to 4 times a day – a total of 8 tablets a day.

- Take marshmallow root powder, especially if there is a burning sensation associated with the diarrhoea (for precautions see page 48). *Adults:* 1 teaspoon of powder mixed with water, 1-3 times a day.

Children (2-16 years old): adjust the adult dose downwards, depending on the age of the child – see Chapter 6.

- Meadowsweet or chamomile tea can be very effective in treating mild diarrhoea in children (for precautions see page 47). *Adults:* 2-4 cups a day. *Children:* 2-5-year-olds: 5-10 teaspoons a day; 6-12-year-olds: 1-2 cups a day; older children: 2-4 cups a day.

ANTI-DIARRHOEA MIX

Ingredients
- 30ml witch hazel leaf tincture (1:2)
- 40ml barberry tincture (1:10) (for precautions see page 51)
- 40ml chamomile tincture (1:5) (for precautions see page 47)

To make
- Mix ingredients together.
- Pour into a clean, dark glass bottle.
- Label with the contents and the date.
- Store at room temperature for up to a year.

Adult dose: 10ml diluted with some water, 2-4 times a day for 1-2 days, then reduce the dose to 5ml, 1-3 times a day, until symptoms improve.

EXCESS WIND

Producing too much wind can be a function of diet (a vegetarian diet with lots of lentils, for instance) or can be related to having the wrong bacteria balance in the gut, which may result from taking lots of antibiotics. Occasionally, specific foods may need to be excluded from the diet. Often, flatulence goes together with indigestion and leads to bloating or colicky pain.

Treatment options

- Drink fennel tea after meals. *Adults:* ½ -1 cup, 1-3 times a day.

- Drink peppermint tea (for precautions see page 48). *Adults:* 1 cup 2 times a day.

- Take aniseed tincture (for precautions see page 50). *Adults:* 1-2 ml diluted with some water, 1-3 times a day, tincture strength 1:2.

- Take probiotics for a month, according to the manufacturer's instructions.

Children (2-16 years old): adjust the adult dose downwards, depending on the age of the child – see Chapter 6.

FOOD INTOLERANCES

Practitioner treatment is recommended for this condition.

These are often incorrectly referred to as food allergies: true food allergies result in much more severe symptoms, including anaphylactic shock. Food intolerance leads to digestive discomfort after eating a particular food type: sometimes headaches, sometimes skin rashes (eczema). Such food sensitivities seem to be very common nowadays.

Herbalists often recommend that you improve your digestive function and the condition of your intestines, rather than exclude half the foods from your diet.

Treatment options

- Supplement with probiotics for a month; take according to the manufacturer's instructions.

- Improve your digestive function by combining a bitter herb with a restorative and a demulcent herb into a tea and drinking it on a daily basis until the symptoms improve. Two examples are given below and overleaf.

TEA FOR REDUCING FOOD INTOLERANCES (NO.1)

Ingredients
- 50g dry vervain
- 50g dry marshmallow leaf
- 50g dry calendula (for precautions see page 114).

To make
- Mix herbs thoroughly.
- Infuse 2 teaspoons of the mix in a cupful of freshly boiled water for 10 minutes. Strain and drink warm. You can add honey to this tea.

Adult dose: 1-2 cups a day, separately from meals.

Children (2-16 years old): adjust the adult dose downwards, depending on the age of the child – see Chapter 6.

TEA FOR REDUCING FOOD INTOLERANCES (NO.2)

Ingredients

- 50g dry barberry (for precautions see page 51)
- 50g dry chamomile (for precautions see page 47)
- 50g dry marshmallow leaf

To make

- Mix herbs thoroughly.
- Infuse 2 teaspoons of the mix in a cupful of freshly boiled water for 10 minutes. Strain and drink warm. You can add honey to this tea.

Adult dose: 1-2 cups a day, separately from meals.

FOOD POISONING

Medical help is strongly advised for this condition.

Food poisoning usually develops rapidly a few hours after eating an offending meal. The usual symptoms include severe stomach ache, nausea, vomiting and, later, diarrhoea. You must seek medical help if the symptoms persist for more than a few hours or are very severe.

Treatment options

- Take charcoal tablets with some water, if you can manage to keep them down! Adults: 2 tablets every 2 hours, up to 8 tablets a day, with plenty of water.
- Drink strong chamomile tea to reduce the stomach irritation (for precautions see page 47). Adults: 1-3 cups a day.

- Resort to the anti-diarrhoea mix (see page 58) if diarrhoea is a prominent feature.

Children (2-16 years old): adjust the adult dose downwards, depending on the age of the child – see Chapter 6.

GALL BLADDER, REMOVED

If you have had your gall bladder removed owing to gallstones, you may experience digestive problems for a while: there may be urgency of bowel movement; looseness of stools; aches and pains in the abdomen. The symptoms are caused by the irritating effect of bile that is released into the digestive tract all the time, even in the absence of food. Make sure you eat little and often, and with each meal have a small amount of food that contains fat (e.g. cheese, meat, fish, salad with a dressing, etc.). The idea is to make use of your bile to digest fat, thus reducing the 'unused' bile which irritates the bowels. You can also drink soothing, demulcent herbs as teas to reduce the irritation.

Treatment options

- Drink chamomile tea (for precautions see page 47). Adults: 1-2 cups a day.

- Drink marshmallow leaf tea. Adults: 1-2 cups a day.

- Take marshmallow root powder (for precautions see page 48). Adults: 1 teaspoon mixed with water, 1-2 times a day.

- Take linseed. Adults: pre-soak 1 tablespoon of linseed in a cup of boiled, cooled water; stir and drink the water with the seeds in the morning.

Children (2-16 years old): adjust the adult dose

downwards, depending on the age of the child – see Chapter 6.

GUM PROBLEMS

If your gums are inflamed or bleeding when you brush your teeth, you may be suffering from early signs of gum disease. A visit to a dentist is a must and you may have to improve your oral hygiene routine. There may be nutritional shortcomings in your diet, and specific supplements may be suggested by a health practitioner.

Treatment options

- Take propolis tablets/capsules for a few weeks; take according to the manufacturer's instructions.

- Use a herbal mouthwash (see below and right) on a daily basis until there is an improvement.

MOUTHWASH MIX (NO.1)

Ingredients
- 30ml sage (tincture strength 1:2)
- 40ml chamomile (tincture strength 1:5) (for precautions see page 47.
- 30ml thyme (tincture strength 1:2)

To make
- Mix ingredients together.
- Pour into a clean, dark glass bottle.
- Label with the contents and the date.
- Store at room temperature for up to a year.

Adults and children over 5 years old: Dilute 1ml of the tincture mix with 30ml of water and swirl around your mouth for about 1 minute, twice a day after brushing your teeth.

MOUTHWASH MIX (NO.2)

Ingredients
- 30ml propolis (tincture strength 1:10) (for precautions see page 99)
- 40ml sage (tincture strength 1:2)
- 30ml calendula (tincture strength 1:2) (for precautions see page 114)

To make
- Mix ingredients together.
- Pour into a clean, dark glass bottle.
- Label with the contents and the date.
- Store at room temperature for up to a year.

Adults and children over 5 years old: Dilute 1ml of the tincture mix with 30ml of water and swirl around your mouth for about 1 minute, twice a day after brushing your teeth.

HAEMORRHOIDS (PILES)

Practitioner treatment is recommended for this condition.

Haemorrhoids are a troublesome problem at the very end of the digestive tract! Make sure you do not get constipated, as that can make the problem worse. If the haemorrhoids don't improve quickly with the external application of the cream described overleaf, you may need an internal treatment from a herbalist.

Treatment options

- Apply a compress of warm calendula tea to the anus 2-5 times a day (use little cotton wool pieces rather than cloth, soak each one thoroughly, hold gently pressed against the haemorrhoids until the tea cools down, and use another piece to repeat the procedure). For precautions see page 114.

- Apply plain calendula cream or ointment to the anus 2 times a day. For precautions see page 114.

CREAM FOR HAEMORRHOIDS

Ingredients
- 25g calendula cream (for precautions see page 114)
- 5ml witch hazel tincture or witch hazel distilled water

To make
- Mix well.
- Transfer to a clean, dark glass jar, making sure that there are no air pockets left. Store for up to 12 months.

To use: apply to the anus twice a day.

Note: this cream may sting temporarily.

HEARTBURN / HIATUS HERNIA / GASTRO-OESOPHAGEAL REFLUX

Practitioner treatment is recommended for this condition.

Caution: If you are pregnant, or suffer from high blood pressure or water retention, you can use liquorice on a one-off basis but do not use it regularly.

Heartburn is a burning pain behind the sternum (breastbone) which results from hiatus hernia or reflux. The pain is caused by stomach acid getting into the oesophagus and irritating its surface. Sometimes this pain causes chest tightness and is similar to that of angina (heart ache), so if you are not sure, check your symptoms with your GP. Heartburn is often related to diet, stress level, lifestyle and being overweight, which all need to be addressed to sort out the problem for good.

Occasionally babies suffer from reflux, but I would not recommend treating this at home.

Treatment options

- Take marshmallow root powder when you experience the symptoms. *Adults:* 1 teaspoon of the powder mixed with some lukewarm water to a 'runny custard' consistency; after you have swallowed it you can follow with a sip of water to take the taste away. Such a marshmallow 'meal' can bring almost instantaneous relief. For precautions see page 48.

- Take liquorice root powder in a similar manner to the marshmallow root powder (for precautions see page 53).

- Drink meadowsweet tea (for precautions see page 47). *Adults:* 1-3 cups a day.

- Drink marshmallow leaf tea. *Adults:* 1-3 cups a day.

- Drink lemon balm tea if your heartburn is related to stress. *Adults:* 1-2 cups a day.

Children (2-16 years old): adjust the adult dose downwards, depending on the age of the child – see Chapter 6.

MOUTH ULCERS

Mouth ulcers result from a number of causes: sometimes they are due to a harsh detergent used in the dishwasher, or not rinsing the dishes properly after washing up; sometimes to a scratch from eating a particular food or brushing your teeth too vigorously. On other occasions the frequent presence of mouth ulcers points towards a weakened immune system or even a serious dysfunction of the digestive system, in which case you should seek professional advice.

Treatment options

All the gargles below are suitable for children over 4 years old.

- Gargle with chamomile tea every hour for 1-2 minutes until you feel an improvement. For precautions see page 47.

- Gargle with calendula tea every hour for 1-2 minutes until you feel an improvement. For precautions see page 114.

- Gargle with sage tea every 2 hours for 1 minute until you feel an improvement.

GARGLE WITH PROPOLIS TINCTURE DILUTED IN WATER

To use
- Dilute 1ml of propolis tincture in 30ml of water (for precautions see page 99).
- Gargle 2-5 times a day, for half a minute. The solution may sting initially.

MORNING SICKNESS

Morning sickness is a name for nausea which affects most women during the first three months of pregnancy. Eating something straight away in the morning before getting up can help a lot (a biscuit, sweet or savoury); so will a cup of warm herbal tea (you can make it the previous evening and keep a thermos by your bed). The herbal teas recommended below should be fairly weak: either use tea bags or reduce the normal brewing time to 1-2 minutes if using dry herbs.

Nausea that persists beyond the first three months of pregnancy needs professional attention.

Treatment options

- Drink ginger tea (use a ginger tea bag, a teaspoon of ginger powder or a slice of fresh ginger per cup of water; add lemon and honey if you wish). For precautions see page 52. *Adults:* 1-3 cups a day.

- Drink chamomile tea (use a chamomile tea bag or a teaspoonful of dry herbs per cup of water). For precautions see page 47. *Adults:* 1-3 cups a day.

NAUSEA

Nausea can accompany many ailments that upset the digestive system. Sometimes it is not related to the digestive system at all – for instance, people with migraines often feel sick, as do people with inner-ear problems. The measures described overleaf refer to feeling sick after eating some suspect food or having a stomach bug.

Treatment options

- Drink peppermint tea (for precautions see page 48). *Adults:* 1-2 cups a day.

- Drink chamomile tea (for precautions see page 47) *Adults:* 1-3 cups a day.

Children (2-16 years old): adjust the adult dose downwards, depending on the age of the child – see Chapter 6.

PREVENTION OF DIGESTIVE PROBLEMS ON HOLIDAY

There are a few simple rules that will help you avoid stomach problems when travelling abroad.

- Don't drink anything but boiled or bottled drinks.

- Don't have any ice in your drinks.

- Avoid salads, and fruit that cannot be peeled.

- Make sure that food is well cooked when eating out.

- Be fastidious about washing your hands after going to the toilet and before handling any food.

Nowadays you can get hand washes that can be used without any water. However, if you are going somewhere exotic and remote you may want to take charcoal tablets and anti-diarrhoea mix (see page 58) with you, just in case.

Preventative measures

- Eat fresh garlic every day (for precautions see page 52). *Adults:* a clove of garlic, crushed and mixed with a teaspoon of honey, 1-2 times a day.

- Take a single dose of charcoal and anti-diarrhoea mix if you have eaten or drunk something that has the potential to cause a problem (see Diarrhoea entry, page 58).

STOMACH ACHE

The good old hot-water bottle applied to the stomach area can often do the trick, especially if the pain is caused by trapped wind. Persistent and severe pain that will not improve with the measures below needs to be checked by a health professional.

Treatment options

- Drink peppermint tea (for precautions see page 48). *Adults:* 1-2 cups a day.

- Drink chamomile tea (for precautions see page 47). *Adults:* 1-3 cups a day.

- Drink lemon balm tea if the ache is caused by stress or anxiety. *Adults:* 1-3 cups a day.

- Take some marshmallow root powder or liquorice root powder if the pain has a burning quality (see Heartburn entry on page 62). For precautions see pages 48 and 53.

Children (2-16 years old): adjust the adult dose downwards, depending on the age of the child – see Chapter 6.

STOMACH ACIDITY – TOO LOW

This condition is difficult to diagnose as it may mimic other conditions. It is usually diagnosed in connection with other health issues, such as food sensitivities or skin problems, so I would advise seeking professional opinion if you suspect it.

Herbalists treat low acidity by stimulating

the production and release of stomach acid with bitter herbs. These must be taken 15-30 minutes before eating and the bitter taste needs to be 'tasted', therefore you need to sip the herbs slowly. You can use either teas or tinctures as long as they taste bitter! Each of the tinctures below can be used by itself, or you can combine any two.

Treatment options

- Drink strong chamomile or vervain tea (for precautions see page 47). *Adults:* 1-2 cups a day, before meals.

- Take dandelion root in a tincture form (for precautions see page 51). *Adults:* 3-5ml, 1-3 times a day, tincture strength 1:5; dilute each dose in half a cup of lukewarm water and sip slowly.

- Take barberry in a tincture form (for precautions see page 51). *Adults:* 2-4ml, 1-3 times a day, tincture strength 1:10; dilute each dose in half a cup of lukewarm water and sip slowly.

- Take hops in a tincture form (for precautions see page 83). *Adults:* 0.5-1ml, 1-3 times a day, tincture strength 1:2; dilute each dose in half a cup of lukewarm water and sip slowly.

Children (2-16 years old): adjust the adult dose downwards, depending on the age of the child – see Chapter 6.

STOMACH ACIDITY – TOO HIGH

Practitioner treatment is recommended for this condition.

This condition is often related to stress. If that is the case it may be worth taking relaxing herbs long-term to deal with the effects of stress (see Chapter 13). There may also be other factors at play, such as diet or genetic predisposition. The common symptoms include heartburn, bloating and stomach pain. Make sure you have a proper diagnosis, rather than treating on the basis of an assumption, as the symptoms of low acidity may be remarkably similar. The measures below will make you more comfortable, but it may be tricky to get rid of the problem for good yourself.

Treatment options

- Drink chamomile and meadowsweet tea, mixed in equal proportions (for precautions see page 47). *Adults:* 3 cups a day, reducing to 1 cup a day once symptoms improve

- Take marshmallow root powder, which will protect the stomach lining from possible damage (for precautions see page 48). *Adults:* 1 teaspoon mixed with ⅓ cup of water, 3 times a day, between meals.

Children (2-16 years old): adjust the adult dose downwards, depending on the age of the child – see Chapter 6.

VOMITING

Vomiting is, in a way, a healthy sign of your body trying to get rid of something harmful. You should not try to suppress it, but allow for plenty of rest and take little sips of either water, ordinary black tea or chamomile tea after you have been sick. The most common reasons for vomiting are food or alcohol poisoning or a 'tummy bug' (usually a viral infection). However, vomiting is not always connected directly with a problem in your stomach – it can be a sign of other diseases, for instance, migraine, concussion, meningitis or inner-ear problems. A baby or a small child that keeps being violently sick should be taken to a doctor without delay, as there is a danger of rapid dehydration.

Treatment options

- Drink weak chamomile tea in small amounts until the symptoms improve; you can give this tea to children a teaspoon at a time. For precautions see page 47.

- Take charcoal if you suspect food poisoning. Even if you are sick after taking the tablets, you will get some benefit as the charcoal dissolves and acts rapidly once swallowed. *Adults:* 2 tablets up to 4 times a day.

Children (2-16 years old): adjust the adult dose downwards, depending on the age of the child – see Chapter 6.

WORMS

Practitioner treatment is recommended for this condition.

The most common worms are threadworms, and the treatment below refers to these. Try the recommended options for a couple of weeks, but if these do not work a herbalist may prescribe stronger worm-killing herbs. It is best not to self-medicate with these, as such herbs, if overdosed, can be potentially harmful.

Treatment options

- Take fresh garlic. *Adults:* 1 chopped clove mixed in a spoonful of honey, 3 times a day. *Children (6-16 years old):* adjust the adult dose downwards, depending on the age of the child – see Chapter 6. Garlic is not suitable for children under 6 years old.

- Eat lots of freshly grated carrots or drink carrot juice every day; do not continue for more then 2 weeks. Note that the skin can become slightly yellow if you drink lots of carrot juice: this is a harmless phenomenon and will disappear when you stop drinking it. *Adults:* 3-4 carrots a day. *Children (2-12 years old):* 1-2 carrots a day.

- Munch on pumpkin seeds through the day. *Adults:* a handful a day. *Children (4-12 years old):* half a handful a day.

WHEN AND WHY YOU SHOULD SEE A PROFESSIONAL MEDICAL HERBALIST

- Irritable bowel syndrome: herbalists recognise many variants of IBS and the treatment will vary accordingly; this individualised approach leads to a very high rate of permanent relief from the symptoms.

- Ulcerative colitis / Crohn's disease: the treatment requires specific protocols of diet and herbs, and, as patients are often on steroids, the treatment needs to be supervised in conjunction with a GP or a consultant gastroenterologist.

- Stomach and duodenal ulcer: these are potentially dangerous conditions that respond remarkably well to herbal treatment: it is possible to combine orthodox and herbal treatment to improve the outcome.

- Liver disease: herbalists can help in many situations; however, it is usually best to work in conjunction with your GP in order to monitor the liver function.

- Gall bladder disease (gallstones): treating gallstones with home remedies can be dangerous, as a gallstone can lodge in the duct leading out of the gall bladder and cause serious complications.

- Diverticulitis: this requires a comprehensive review of diet and lifestyle as well as the use of individually appropriate herbs.

- Stomach or bowel cancer: herbalists are not allowed to treat cancer without the agreement of the patient's doctor, but they can often offset the side effects of the orthodox treatment.

THE FOLLOWING SYMPTOMS WARRANT SEEING A HEALTH PROFESSIONAL WITHOUT DELAY

- Persistent, intense pain in the abdomen.

- Blood in the stools (this will look red if the bleeding occurs from the lower digestive tract, but if the bleeding comes from the upper digestive tract it will look like coffee grains in the stools, or the stools will become black).

- Stomach pain and/or diarrhoea and running a high temperature.

- A radical change in your bowel habit without any obvious reason, or one which persists.

- Your child becomes 'floppy' after being repeatedly sick or having bad diarrhoea – he or she may be dangerously dehydrated.

Chapter 12
The muscular and skeletal systems

The muscular system consists of all the muscles and ligaments in your body that are attached to the bones. Your heart and the smooth muscles that are present in the digestive and circulatory systems are also muscle tissues, but usually cannot voluntarily be controlled. The skeletal system comprises all the bones, including the skull and the spine, as well as all the joints that articulate the bones. Because the muscular and skeletal systems are so intimately connected it makes sense to discuss them together.

SAFETY AND COMPATIBILITY

Many common problems associated with joints and muscles can be safely treated at home, and herbs can offer a lot in terms of pain and inflammation control. However, some of the recommended remedies need to be used in a specific way, otherwise they can be potentially harmful (for example, arnica). Some remedies may not be compatible with conventional medication for joint disorders. In the latter case, a medical herbalist may advise you on alternative herbs that can work alongside the orthodox medication –it is generally not safe to try such remedies yourself.

Herbalists can also offset the side effects of medication used for the treatment of advanced arthritis.

OTHER THERAPIES

There are many complementary therapies that deal with joint and muscle problems, especially back problems. Herbal medicine works extremely well in conjunction with such therapies, for example, osteopathy, and I would encourage you to combine herbs with another therapy of your choice to deal with problems that are 'mechanical' in nature, such as strain injuries, misalignment, bad posture and so on.

SUPPLEMENTS

Both the muscular and skeletal systems often benefit from specific supplementation that aids the rate of healing and reduces inflammatory tendencies. The need for such supplementation should be individually assessed by a specialist in view of your age, lifestyle and diet. Medical herbalists can advise you on both the appropriate herbal remedies and nutritional measures.

MUST-HAVE HERBS

The herbs in this section are arranged in order of usefulness.

ARNICA

Warning: For external use only. Do not apply to open skin injuries.

Caution needed if allergic to plants of the *Compositae* family.

Uses

This herb provides the best treatment for bruising and should be used only in cream or ointment form. Any bumps, knocks or sprains, if treated immediately with arnica, will have minimal swelling and bruising and will heal much quicker. It is a fantastic treatment for children when they bump their heads – a quick application of arnica cream to the injured spot (as long as the skin is not broken) will ease the pain within minutes, and there will be no blue bump either. I have used it on fingers trapped in doors, toes crushed by heavy stones, innumerable bumps on the head and swollen knees after skiing – always with amazing results.

How to apply

Arnica is not suitable for internal use as it can be quite toxic, unless it is in a homeopathic form. For the same reason you should not apply it to open wounds and cuts, as too much arnica can then be absorbed into the bloodstream. However, applying the ointment well away from the cut is acceptable: keep a 2-3cm gap between the margin of the cut and the cream application, and apply arnica in a thinner layer than you would to unbroken skin, where it can be applied quite liberally. There is little point in applying arnica to injuries that are more than one day old – arnica is very much a first-aid item that must be applied as **soon as possible** after the injury to prevent local haemorrhage and swelling.

How often

Normally, one generous application is sufficient to prevent bruise formation, but some injuries (for instance, swollen knees due to excessive exercise) will benefit from 2-3 applications every 2-3 hours.

Suitability

Arnica cream is suitable for all group ages, including babies, and for pregnant women as long as it is applied to unbroken skin.

COMFREY

Warning: Use only for external treatment.

Uses

This is another herb that should be used only externally unless under the guidance of a medical herbalist. It is a great healer for fractures, sprains, a bad back and even broken bones! The old name for comfrey is 'knitbone', as it was used in the past to aid the healing of broken bones. Comfrey ointment or a poultice can be applied to sprained ankles, swollen knees, broken ribs, the collarbone or fingers (as they cannot be put in plaster). This is a herb that I would choose to apply to so-called 'mixed wounds' (bruising and cuts to the skin) instead of arnica, and a herb that 'takes over' from arnica to aid recovery from the injury. Comfrey ointment/cream provides the best base for customising your remedy with the addition of different essential oils and tinctures.

How to apply

The type of external application of comfrey should be dictated by the type of injury: if there is a lot of recent swelling, choose a compress or poultice; if it is a long-term treatment, go for the cream or ointment.

How often

The frequency of application (irrespective of the type) depends on the injury: the more recent the injury, the more often you should apply the treatment (3-5 times a day); for a long-term problem apply the treatment 1-2 times a day.

Suitability
Comfrey is safe for external use for all age groups, including babies, and for pregnant women.

CRAMP BARK

Uses
Cramp bark is a muscular relaxant, therefore it is suitable for problems where muscles go into spasm or become tense. It will help with muscular pain that is secondary to nerve pain, for instance in sciatica, or when muscle tension leads to neck pain or tension headache. Cramp bark is also useful for smooth muscle tension and can be used for stomach cramps caused by IBS.

How to use
As tincture, either added to ointments or taken internally.

How often
Ointments with cramp bark can be applied 2-3 times a day until the symptoms improve.

Dosage
Adults: 0.7-1.3ml diluted with some water, 1-3 times a day, tincture strength 1:2.
Children (2-16 years old): adjust the adult dose downwards, depending on the age of the child – see Chapter 6.

WILLOW BARK

Caution needed if allergic to salicylate compounds. Best avoided when breastfeeding.

Uses
Willow bark has been used for rheumatic complaints for centuries. The salicylic acid compounds in the willow bark extract are responsible for its anti-inflammatory and pain-killing actions, and it was salicylic acid itself that was a precursor to modern-day aspirin. Willow bark extract can be used in any muscular or joint ailments that are inflammatory in nature and manifest themselves as pain or swelling. It is the best treatment for back pain, whether of recent origin or long-standing. Recommendations for using willow bark include any type of arthritis, inflammation of the joints, muscle ache (especially if secondary to joint ache), muscle tension and tension headache.

Purple willow (*Salix purpurea*) products are superior to white willow (*Salix alba*) products, but not easy to acquire.

Combinations
Willow bark combines well with other anti-rheumatic and anti-inflammatory remedies such as wild yam, liquorice and celery seed.

How to use
The tincture can be added directly to the anti-inflammatory ointments (5ml per 20g of cream) or taken internally. In my experience the tincture dosage needed for the anti-inflammatory and analgesic effect to be taken internally is quite high and may prove tricky to achieve (willow bark extract has an unpleasant

strong taste); therefore I would recommend the tablets made from the freeze-dried extract.

Dosage

Adults: 1-4 tablets a day (each tablet should provide the equivalent of 8g of dried herb); or 1-2.3ml diluted with some water, 1-3 times a day, tincture strength 1:2 – if you are brave enough to tackle the taste!

Children (2-16 years old): adjust the adult dose downwards, depending on the age of the child – see Chapter 6.

ROSEMARY

Warning: Do not use essential oils for external applications in pregnancy or for children under 3 years old without consulting a specialist.

Uses

This herb is good for all sorts of muscular pain. It will help to relax and soothe aching muscles after heavy exercise or when suffering from a cold. It will also warm the muscles, by stimulating the circulation to them, and reduce muscular tension.

How to use

As rosemary essential oil. Put it in a bath or add to the creams or ointments.

Dosage

Adults: 5 drops of essential oil in a bath, once a day; or 10 drops of essential oil to 50g of comfrey cream, apply 1-3 times a day.

Children (3-16 years old): adjust the adult dose downwards, depending on the age of the child – see Chapter 6.

OPTIONAL HERBS

CELERY SEED

Caution needed if you have kidney disorders or when breastfeeding.

Uses

Celery seed has a wide range of applications for the muscular and skeletal systems: gout, osteoarthritis, rheumatoid arthritis, rheumatic pains and muscular aches. This herb is one of the herbal detoxifiers, mainly through its diuretic action. Celery seed extract helps to eliminate metabolic waste products from the blood which, if not removed effectively, can cause the aggravation of joint inflammation.

Combinations

It combines well with liquorice, wild yam and willow bark.

How to take

As tincture.

Dosage

Adults: 1.5-3ml diluted with some water, 1-3 times a day, tincture strength 1:2. Remember to drink plenty of water to make up for the diuretic action of the herb.

Children (2-16 years old): adjust the adult dose downwards, depending on the age of the child – see Chapter 6.

Chilli (cayenne pepper)

Warning: Do not apply to broken skin.
Avoid contact with the eyes.
Do not use for acute inflammation such as a gout attack.

Uses

Cayenne pepper is useful for rheumatic complaints chiefly on account of its ability to numb the local nerves (analgesic action) and increase the local blood supply. The latter action helps to 'flush' a specific area free of the accumulated waste products or allergenic substances which often cause joint problems. The addition of chilli tincture to a healing cream will speed up recovery after an injury involving extensive bruising. Make sure you wash your hands well after applying the cream. Chillies will not cause any harm in spite of the stinging; wash with cold water if necessary.

How to use

As tincture added to comfrey cream.

Dosage

Adults and children above 3 years old:
Add no more than 10 drops of the chilli tincture (strength 1:3) to 50g of the cream/ointment base (if the cream stings after the application you have added too much). I would avoid this cream in small children as they are likely to transfer the cream accidentally to the eyes.

Lavender

Warning: Do not use essential oils for external applications in pregnancy or for children under 3 years old without consulting a specialist.

Uses

Lavender can help with a variety of rheumatic and post-traumatic pains, for instance after a fall. It is gently relaxing for the muscles and will therefore help with any muscle tension or a spasm caused by the inflammation or injury. It is also anti-inflammatory and anti-rheumatic. I recommend adding it to the healing creams that deal with extensive bruising or non-specific rheumatic pains.

How to use

As lavender essential oil added to comfrey cream.

Dosage

Adults and children: 10 drops of lavender essential oil to 50g of the cream base (e.g. comfrey cream).

Meadowsweet

Caution needed if allergic to salicylates. Seek professional advice if pregnant or breastfeeding.

Uses

Meadowsweet is a gentle anti-inflammatory due to its salicylate compounds. As it is a digestive agent as well, it is most suitable for those whose stomach suffers from taking conventional anti-inflammatory medication.

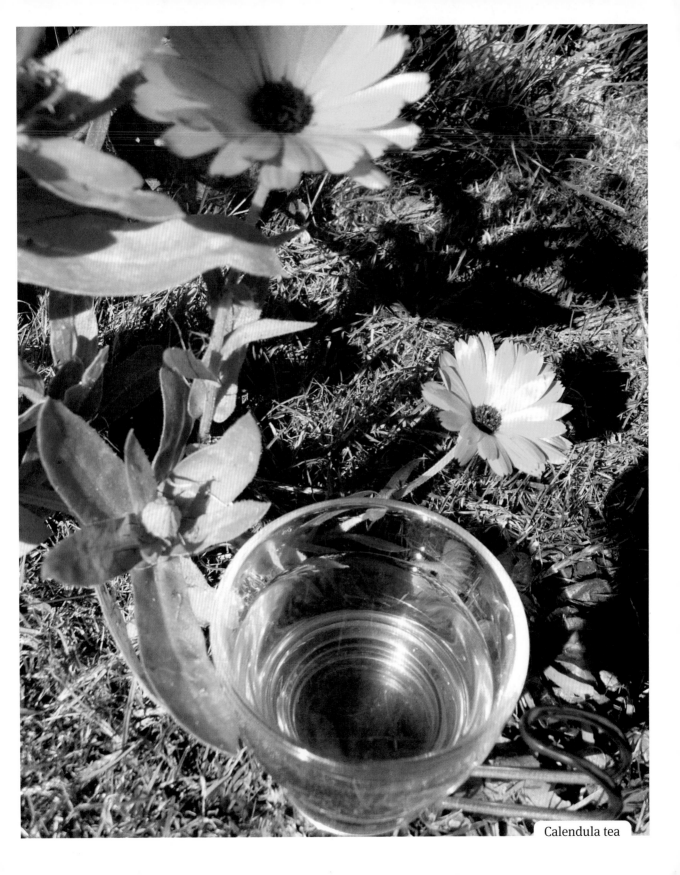

Calendula tea

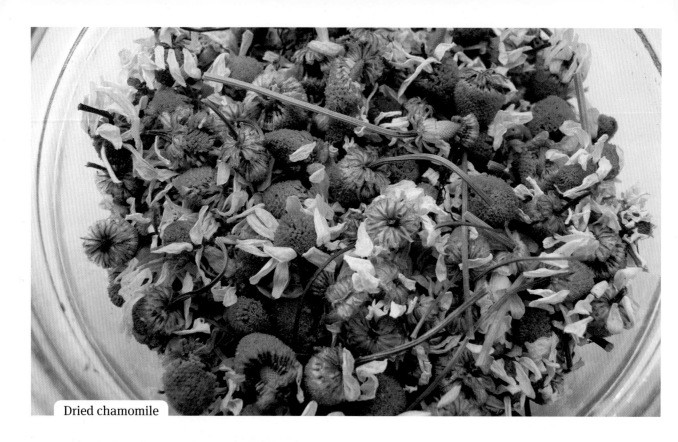

Dried chamomile

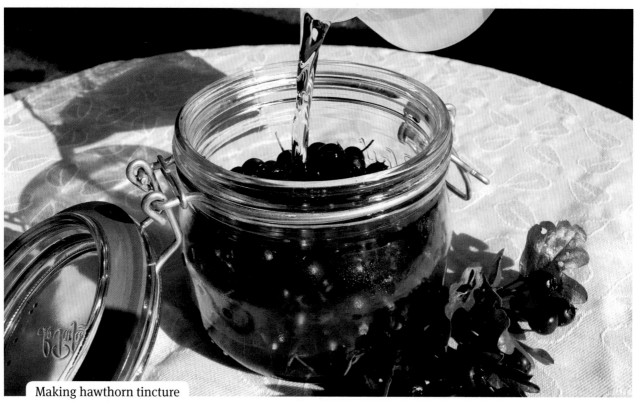

Making hawthorn tincture

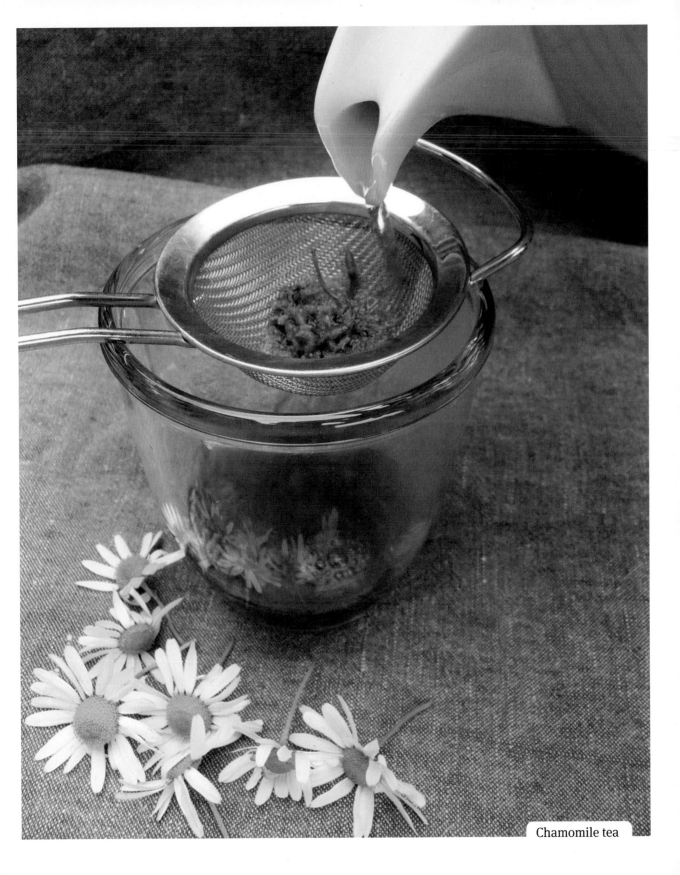

Chamomile tea

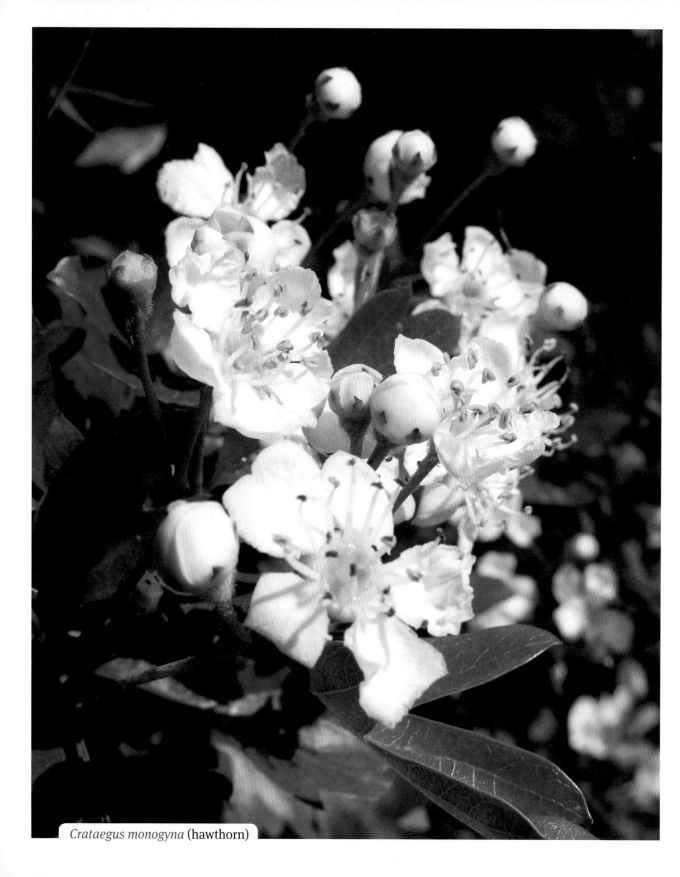

Crataegus monogyna (hawthorn)

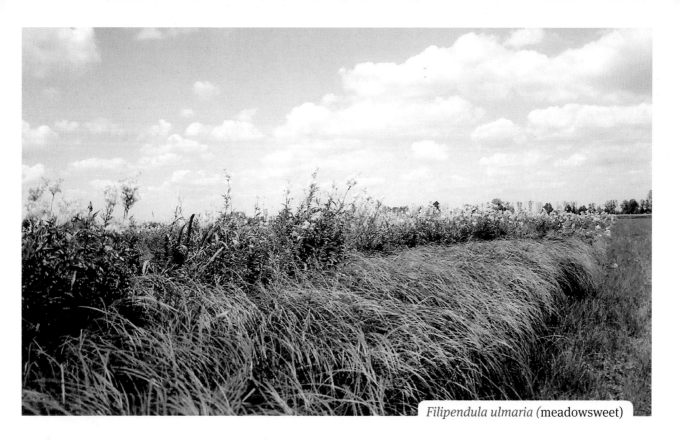

Filipendula ulmaria (meadowsweet)

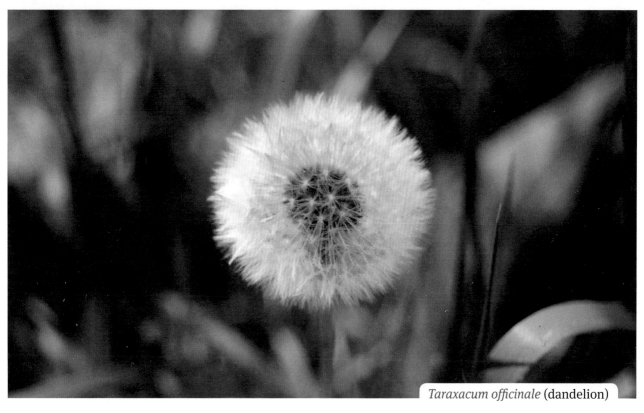

Taraxacum officinale (dandelion)

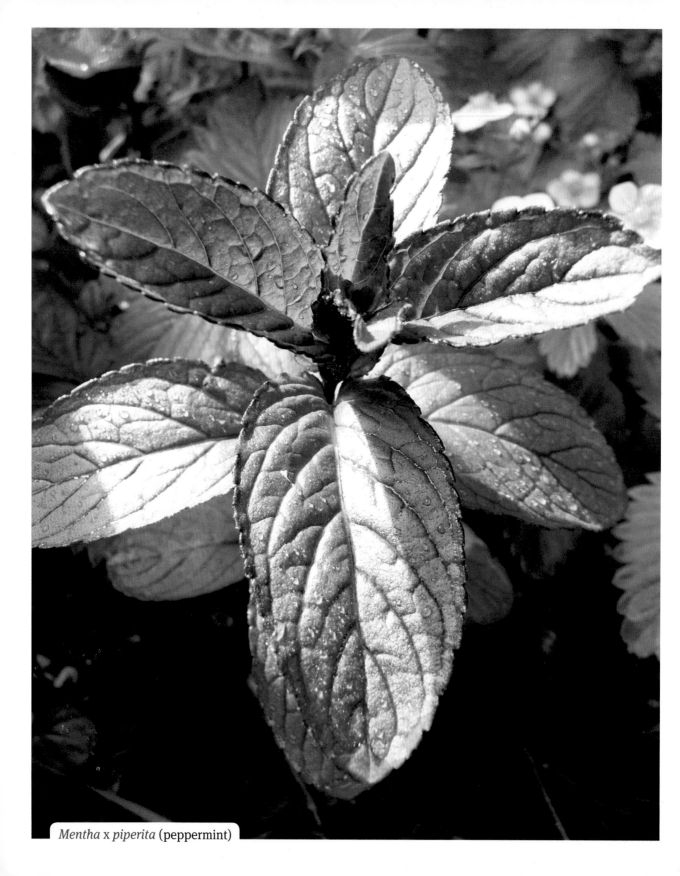

Mentha x *piperita* (peppermint)

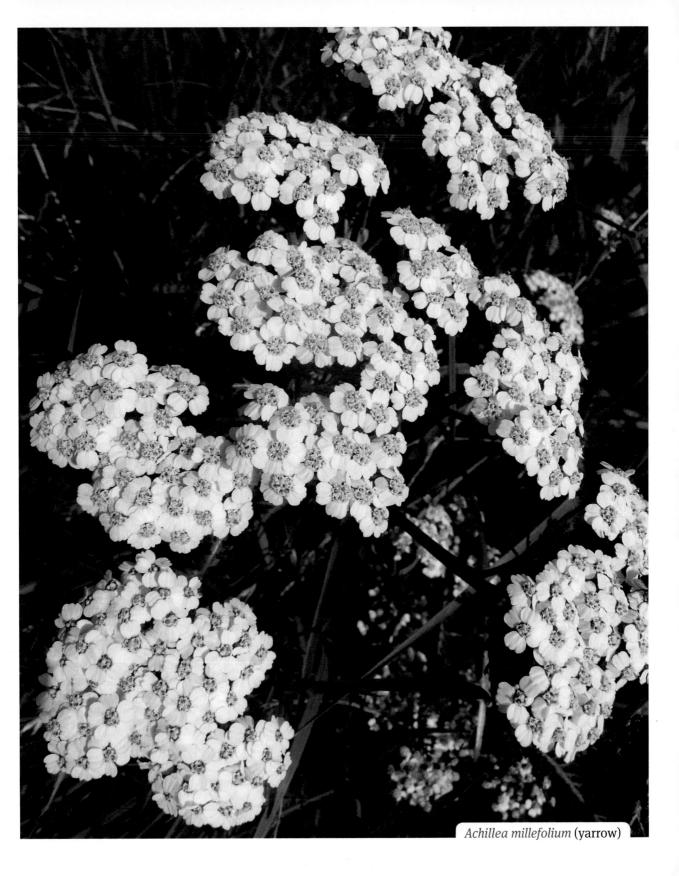

Achillea millefolium (yarrow)

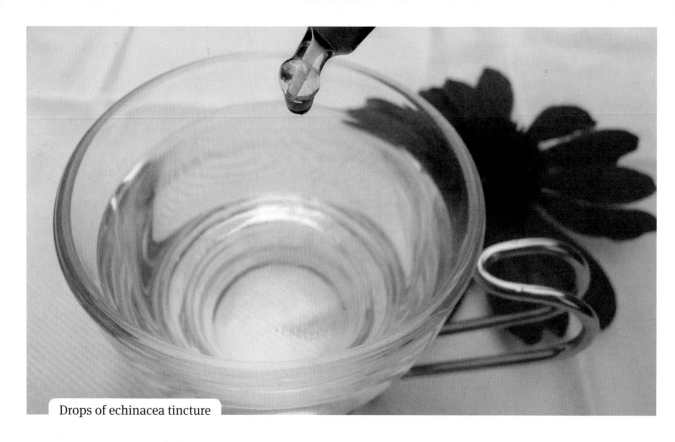

Drops of echinacea tincture

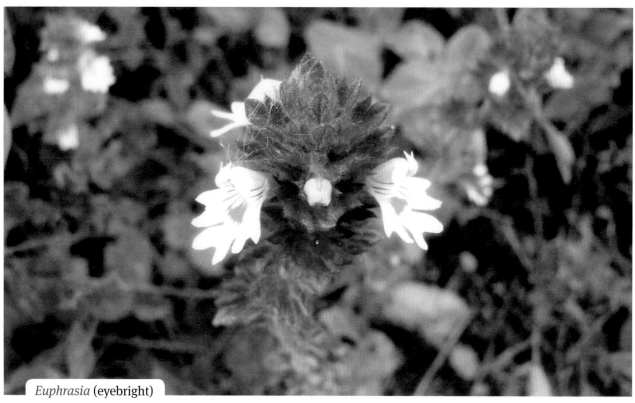

Euphrasia (eyebright)

How to take

I suggest taking it as a tea as an additional treatment for any joint/muscle pain.

Dosage

Adults: 1-2 cups a day.

Children (2-16 years old): adjust the adult dose downwards, depending on the age of the child – see Chapter 6.

NETTLE LEAF

Uses

Nettle, being a detoxifying and anti-allergic herb, has a place in the treatment of joint problems. Such problems often result from bad diet and exposure to environmental allergens, therefore nettle tea provides a logical supportive treatment in most cases.

How to take

As tea or tincture.

Dosage

Adults: 1-2 cups of nettle tea a day; or 0.7-2ml diluted with some water, 2-3 times a day, tincture strength 1:2.

Children (2-16 years old): adjust the adult dose downwards, depending on the age of the child – see Chapter 6.

PEPPERMINT

Warning: Do not use essential oils for external applications in pregnancy or for children under 3 years old without consulting a specialist.

Uses

Peppermint applied externally has cooling and muscle-relaxing properties. These are invaluable where there is pain due to inflammation and/or muscle spasm.

How to use

As peppermint essential oil added to any cream dealing with a recent injury (bruising after a fall, back strain, sprains, etc.) or for providing a gentle analgesic action.

Dosage

Adults and children: Add 5-10 drops of the peppermint essential oil to 50g of a base cream.

BIRCH

Caution needed if allergic to salicylates.

Uses

Birch is anti-arthritic, anti-inflammatory and detoxifying. It is used for all types of arthritis, including gout, especially if there is substantial swelling involved.

Combinations

It can be combined with any other anti-rheumatic remedies.

How to take

As tincture.

Dosage

Adults: 0.7-1.3ml diluted with some water, 2-3 times a day, tincture strength 1:2.

Children (2-16 years old): adjust the adult dose downwards, depending on the age of the child – see Chapter 6.

TURMERIC

Caution needed if taking blood-thinning drugs.

Uses
Turmeric – a familiar spice with its bright yellow colour – is one of the few general herbal anti-inflammatories. It is used internally in cases of osteoarthritis, rheumatoid arthritis and back pain triggered by a variety of various causes.

Combinations
It combines well with wild yam and willow bark.

How to take
As tincture.

Dosage
Adults: 1.5-3ml diluted with some water, 2-3 times a day, tincture strength 1:1.
Children (2-16 years old): adjust the adult dose downwards, depending on the age of the child – see Chapter 6.

WILD YAM

Uses
Wild yam tincture has anti-rheumatic and anti-inflammatory properties. It is useful above all for joint problems that often accompany the menopause, ranging from rheumatoid arthritis to non-specific general joint aches.

Combinations
It combines well with liquorice, celery seed and willow bark.

How to take
As tincture.

Dosage
Adults: 1-2ml diluted with some water, 1-3 times a day, tincture strength 1:2.
Children (2-16 years old): adjust the adult dose downwards, depending on the age of the child – see Chapter 6.

WINTERGREEN

Warning: Do not use essential oils for external applications in pregnancy or for children under 3 years old without consulting a specialist.

Uses
This small evergreen bush yields an essential oil which has a warming and anti-inflammatory effect when applied to the skin around a painful joint.

How to use
As wintergreen essential oil added to comfrey cream.

Dosage
Adults and children: Add 10 drops of the wintergreen essential oil to 50g of comfrey cream and apply to the affected areas 2-3 times a day.

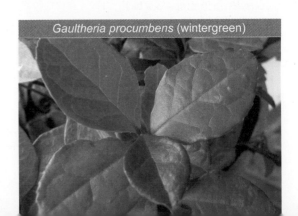
Gaultheria procumbens (wintergreen)

SPECIFIC AILMENTS OF THE MUSCULAR AND SKELETAL SYSTEMS & HERBS THAT CAN HELP

BACK PAIN

All sorts of back pain can be eased with herbal remedies. I follow the school of providing a warm treatment (a bath with essential oils or warming ointment) combined with anti-inflammatory remedies.

Treatment options

- Apply arnica ointment – this should be your first line of treatment following an injury or strain to the back, and should be done as soon as possible. For precautions see page 68. *Adults and children:* apply **once** liberally to the painful area as long as the skin is unbroken. Repeat in a few hours if the injury was extensive.

- Apply comfrey ointment some time after the arnica ointment, or in the first place if it is an open injury. *Adults and children:* keep applying every few hours until there is an improvement.

- Take a hot bath with added essential oils of rosemary or lavender or wintergreen (for precautions see pages 71, 72 and 74). *Adults:* 5-10 drops per bath.

- Take willow bark tablets (for precautions see page 70). *Adults:* Take the maximum dose for a day, according to the manufacturer's instructions, then reduce to the medium dose until the pain eases out.

Children (2-16 years old): adjust the adult dose

downwards, depending on the age of the child – see Chapter 6.

- Apply the cream for muscular tension/spasm (see box below).

> ### CREAM FOR MUSCULAR TENSION/SPASM
> Ingredients
> - 5ml cramp bark (tincture strength 1:2)
> - 20g comfrey cream
>
> To make
> - Mix well.
> - Transfer to a clean, dark glass jar, making sure that there are no air pockets left. Store for up to 12 months.
>
> Adults and children: apply to the affected muscles 2-3 times a day.

BRUISING

Bruising results from varying degrees of bleeding under the skin following an injury. It can also follow any surgical procedure, and can be internal and not obvious on the surface of the skin. Spontaneous bruising that occurs without any injury is a circulatory disorder and should be investigated.

Treatment options

- Arnica ointment/cream is the best treatment – the quicker it is applied the better the result. It is definitely an item to keep in your first-aid kit, both at home and on holiday. It is safe to use on small children, provided the skin is not broken. You can use arnica around a surgical incision to reduce bruising, but leave a good gap of 3-4cm between the application of the ointment and the wound. For precautions see page 68. *Adults and children:* apply it **once** as soon as possible to the injured site.

- If the skin is broken, comfrey cream/ointment is a better all-round remedy as it speeds the healing of both bruises and cuts. *Adults and children:* apply 1-3 times a day, until the bruised area is no longer painful to touch.

FRACTURES

Fractured bones obviously require the attention of a doctor or the emergency services in a hospital. Most cases will end up in plaster, so you will not have much access to the actual site of the fracture. However, you can apply a herbal cream or ointment to the skin adjacent to the plaster, as enough will be absorbed in the area to speed up healing.

In some situations it is not possible to put bones in plaster – for instance if you break your ribs, a finger or toe – in which case you can apply the external treatment directly to the skin over the injured part to speed up the recovery.

Treatment options

- If the skin is intact, apply arnica ointment to the area over the broken bone before the plaster is put on (for precautions see page 68). *Adults and children:* apply **once**, liberally.

- Apply a comfrey poultice or ointment to the area immediately adjacent to the plaster. *Adults and children:* apply once or twice a day for as long as you have the plaster on.

- Apply comfrey ointment directly to the skin over the broken rib, toe or finger – be very gentle. *Adults and children:* twice a day.

GOUT

> Practitioner treatment is recommended for this condition.

The symptoms of gout are swelling of the joint, shiny red skin around the joint and severe pain. The cause is the accumulation of uric acid crystals in the joint, which leads to sudden inflammation. The treatment options below will help to reduce the pain of acute attacks, but to treat recurrent gout you should consult a medical herbalist. Do not put any warming herbs on gout as they can make the inflammation worse.

Treatment options

- For an immediate relief of gout pain use a fresh cabbage leaf poultice: bash a couple of leaves with a rolling pin until some juice appears on the surface or mash the leaves up in a food processor, put the leaves or the mash on a bit of plastic and wrap around the affected joint; keep in place with an elastic bandage. *Adults only:* apply as many times as you need to achieve pain relief, each time keep the poultice in place for half an hour to an hour.

- Drinking celery seed and nettle tea can help to prevent frequent attacks – see box opposite.

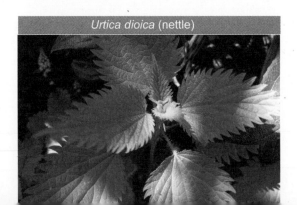
Urtica dioica (nettle)

- Use the cream for painful joints described overleaf.

TEA TO HELP THE FREQUENT RECURRENCE OF GOUT

Ingredients
- 50g dry celery seed (for precautions see page 71)
- 50g dry nettle leaf

To make
- Mix herbs thoroughly.
- Infuse 2 teaspoons of the mix in a cupful of freshly boiled water for 10 minutes. Strain and drink warm. You can add honey to this tea.

Adult dose only: 1 cup a day for many months.

ANTI-RHEUMATIC MIX

Ingredients
- 40ml wild yam (tincture strength 1:2)
- 20ml liquorice (tincture strength 1:1) (for precautions see page 53).
- 20ml celery seed (tincture strength 1:2) (for precautions see page 71)
- 20ml willow bark (tincture strength 1:2) (for precautions see page 70)

To make
- Mix ingredients together.
- Pour into a clean, dark glass bottle.
- Label with the contents and the date.
- Store at room temperature for up to a year.

Adults: 5ml diluted with some water, 2-3 times a day.

Children (2-16 years old): adjust the adult dose downwards, depending on the age of the child – see Chapter 6.

JOINT PAIN

It is difficult to give general advice for joint pain as it may have many causes, so it is often best to see a health professional to get a good diagnosis. However, there are many anti-inflammatory herbs that can be safely tried at home for a variety of joint pains.

Treatment options

- Apply comfrey ointment externally. *Adults and children:* 2-3 times a day.

- Apply a warming chilli cream: add no more than 10 drops of chilli tincture (strength 1:3) to 50g of the cream/ointment base. I would avoid this cream in small children as they are likely to transfer the cream accidentally to the eyes. *Adults and children over 3 years old:* Apply 2-3 times a day to a painful joint.

- A general anti-rheumatic mix can be tried – see box, right.

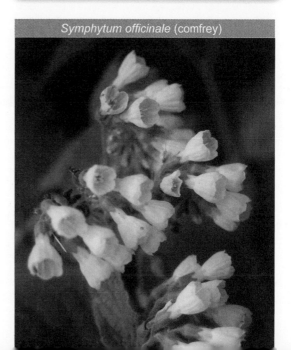

Symphytum officinale (comfrey)

CREAM FOR PAINFUL JOINTS

Ingredients
- 50g comfrey cream
- 5 drops wintergreen essential oil (for precautions see page 74)
- 5 drops lavender essential oil (for precautions see page 72)
- 5 drops peppermint essential oil (for precautions see page 73)

To make
- Mix well.
- Transfer to a clean, dark glass jar, making sure that there are no air pockets left.
- Store for up to 12 months.

Adults and children over 3 years old: Apply to the affected areas 2-3 times a day.

MUSCLE CRAMPS

Muscle cramps can result from a magnesium deficiency, so supplementing with magnesium for a while may bring about a quick improvement. Otherwise muscle-relaxing herbs can be used.

Treatment options

- Take cramp bark tincture, especially if cramping is related to intensive exercise. *Adults:* 0.7-1.3ml diluted with some water, 1-3 times a day, tincture strength 1:2.

- Add muscle-relaxing essential oils, e.g. lavender or rosemary, to the bath (for precautions see pages 72 and 71). *Adults*: 5 drops per bath.

Children (3-16 years old): adjust the adult dose downwards, depending on the age of the child – see Chapter 6.

MUSCULAR PAIN

Muscles can ache after intensive use or if you are suffering from flu or a cold.

Sometimes muscle pain is caused by an underlying condition, e.g. fibromyalgia. In most cases warming baths that stimulate circulation are helpful; in addition, you can take a general anti-inflammatory herb and herbal circulatory stimulants.

Treatment options

- Add rosemary and wintergreen essential oils to your bath (for precautions see pages 71 and 74). *Adults:* 5 drops of either, or 2 drops of each if using them together.

- Take tincture of turmeric (for precautions see page 74). *Adults:* 1.5-3ml diluted with some water, 2-3 times a day, tincture strength 1:1.

Children (3-16 years old): adjust the adult dose downwards, depending on the age of the child – see Chapter 6.

- Take circulatory improvers, e.g. ginger, yarrow, hawthorn or chillies, either as a tea or as a tincture (see Chapter 10 for herbs for the circulatory system).

SPRAINS

With sprains, as with bruising, the sooner you apply the treatment, the better the results. Immediate treatment will diminish the pain and swelling, minimise the development of bruising and speed up the rate of healing. Even if you can't administer a treatment straight away, it is worth using the herbs to aid recovery. Keep on applying the herbal ointment or compress until the symptoms improve.

Treatment options

- Apply arnica ointment (for precautions see page 68). *Adults and children:* apply **once** immediately after the injury, and repeat a few hours later.

- Apply comfrey ointment. *Adults and children:* apply 2-3 times a day until the symptoms improve.

- Apply a warm comfrey poultice or compress from diluted tincture or a strong infusion. *Adults and children:* apply 2-3 times a day until the symptoms improve.

WHEN AND WHY YOU SHOULD SEE A PROFESSIONAL MEDICAL HERBALIST

- Osteoarthritis: many cases of osteoarthritis respond very well to herbal treatment; it does tends to need an ongoing treatment, however, so it is best to have a prescription adjusted for long-term use.

- Rheumatoid arthritis: this is an autoimmune disorder that needs an individualised treatment and often involves a slow adjustment of conventional medication.

- Gout: this is often brought on by specific medication or the wrong diet; a good look at the whole state of health of the sufferer is needed.

- Restless leg syndrome: this can be related to stress, poor circulation and dietary deficiencies; it therefore requires a comprehensive treatment plan.

- Ankylosing spondylitis: this is another autoimmune disorder, which often improves remarkably with the adjustment of diet combined with individual prescription.

- Fibromyalgia: this is a complex disorder of the immune system with muscle pain being a prominent symptom; it requires a complex and long-term treatment.

- Juvenile arthritis: this is a type of rheumatoid arthritis that affects young children; excellent results have been achieved with individualised herbal treatment.

THE FOLLOWING SYMPTOMS WARRANT SEEING A HEALTH PROFESSIONAL WITHOUT DELAY

- Severe joint pain that is progressively getting worse.

- Headache following substantial injury to the head.

- Severe back pain that is getting worse.

- Any severe pain and swelling following a fall (possibility of a fracture).

- Widespread joint and/or muscle ache with a feeling of general malaise persisting for some time.

Chapter 13

The nervous system

The nervous system consists of the brain, the spinal cord and the network of nerve cells throughout the whole body. Disorders of the nervous system are often very complicated. The nervous system is our 'control system', which means that the dysfunction of any body organ or tissue may have its causes in the dysfunction of the nervous system. Herbalists stress the importance of treating both body and mind simultaneously, which reflects the intimate connection of the nervous system with every aspect of our body function.

SYMPTOMS AND HORMONAL INFLUENCES

Ailments affecting the nervous system can manifest in many ways: for instance as a pain or as an altered mood. The hormonal changes in the body may have a profound effect on the nervous system and vice versa, and these two systems frequently need to be treated together. A familiar example of hormonal influence on the nervous system is premenstrual syndrome (PMS).

LENGTH OF TREATMENT

There are many herbs that have beneficial effects on the nervous system and nervous tissue. I would like to stress the restorative function of herbs in relation to this system: some herbs have the capacity to aid the recovery of the nervous system from the effects of stress, illness or accident. Nervous tissue recovers slowly, so treatment of problems relating to the nervous system tends to be long-term – 6-12 months or even longer is not unusual.

NON-ADDICTIVE TREATMENT

The biggest advantage of using herbs as opposed to conventional drugs in the case of the nervous system is that herbs are non-addictive. Many commonly prescribed types of medication for anxiety or sleep problems can lead to a dependency on the drug within a few weeks, and it often takes a very long time to come off such medication. This is not a problem with medicinal herbs, because the mode of action is complex and involves many constituents.

VARIATION IN DOSAGE

It is also worth pointing out that the nervous system tends to respond to herbal remedies in an individual way. Some people may need 5 drops of a sleep mix while others may need 2 teaspoonsful to achieve the same effect. Most people will relax after taking valerian, but a tiny proportion will get anxious or over-animated. You may need to experiment a little to find which herbs and which dosage suit your system. I recommend in general starting with a lower dosage and increasing it if you do not see any improvement.

MIXING HERBS AND CONVENTIONAL MEDICATION

Many of the herbs described below can be taken alongside orthodox medication or used to help in coming off it, but I would strongly advise you to see a medical herbalist to make the best choices.

MUST-HAVE HERBS

The herbs in this section are arranged in order of usefulness.

VALERIAN

Uses

Valerian is a general relaxant for the nerves. It forms the basis of many over-the-counter remedies that help with sleep or anxiety. It can be used in many situations: for instance, when you have problems sleeping, when you are nervous before an exam or job interview, or when you feel stressed at work. It can be employed for older children in some cases of hyperactivity, but the dosage should be adjusted by a herbalist (too much valerian can have a stimulating effect). Valerian takes the edge off anxiety and works quite quickly – normally you should feel more relaxed within half an hour of taking a dose. It can also be used to lessen certain kinds of pain: tension headache, earache or period pain.

Combinations

Valerian works very well on its own, but also combines well with other anti-anxiety or sleep-inducing herbs.

How to take

A tincture is the best way to take this herb. In my experience the dosage can vary a lot depending on how sensitive a particular individual is. My general advice is to try the minimum dose to begin with, but if you don't notice the effect after half an hour take another minimum dose. Next time you use valerian you can try the larger dose straight away. If you feel tired after a dose, you have taken too much (unless you use it as a sleep remedy). I recommend that you use a concentrated tincture: 1:1 strength.

Dosage

Adults: 0.3-1ml diluted with some water, 1-3 times a day, tincture strength 1:1. A larger dose can be taken as a one-off. The specific amounts are given when particular ailments are discussed.

Children (2-16 years old): adjust the adult dose downwards, depending on the age of the child – see Chapter 6.

LAVENDER

Warning: Do not use essential oils for external applications in pregnancy or for children under 3 years old without consulting a specialist.

Uses

Lavender works through its lovely scent, which has a calming and relaxing effect on the mind. It can induce deep sleep and can be safely used with children who become overexcited at bedtime.

How to take

Lavender is best used in the form of an essential oil, either in a bath, directly applied to your pillow or in a vaporiser. You can also take a lavender tea.

Dosage

Adults: 5 drops in a bath; 2-3 drops on a pillow; 1-2 drops in a vaporiser; or 1 cup of lavender tea (use 1 teaspoon of herbs per cup of water).
Children (3-16 years old): adjust the adult dose downwards, depending on the age of the child – see Chapter 6.

ROSEMARY

Warning: Do not use essential oils for external applications in pregnancy or for children under 3 years old without consulting a specialist.

Uses

Rosemary is the opposite of the two herbs described above. It is invigorating and stimulating to the nervous system, and it improves concentration and clarity of mind.

How to take

Rosemary's effect on the brain is through the sense of smell, therefore essential oil is the best way to use it. If you need to revive your energy after a long day, or need to be extra-switched-on in the morning, try a few drops of rosemary essential oil in your bath or shower tray. Sniffing a fresh twig of rosemary will also work – rub it with your fingers to release the scent. If I have a long drive ahead I often put a few fresh twigs of rosemary in my car to help me stay alert.

Dosage

Adults: 5 drops in the bath; or 1-2 drops in a vaporiser.
Children (3-16 years old): adjust the adult dose downwards, depending on the age of the child – see Chapter 6.

CHAMOMILE

Caution needed if allergic to plants of the *Compositae* family.

Uses

Chamomile, being an extremely versatile herb, has many applications in conditions related to the nervous system. Taken before bed, chamomile tea can have a relaxing effect and help you to fall asleep. If you feel stressed, it will calm you down. When your digestion is suffering because of anxiety, chamomile will improve it. It is the best herb to use for children, even small babies, to induce a peaceful sleep or treat the tummy ache that anxious children often suffer from.

How to take

For adults, use a strong chamomile tea made with 2 tea bags or two heaped teaspoonsful of loose herbs per cup of water. For children and babies, use a weak infusion made with 1 tea bag or one small teaspoonful of loose herbs per cup of water, infused for 1 minute. Babies should be given only a tiny amount of weak chamomile tea.

Dosage

Adults: 1 cup of tea as needed, up to 4 cups a day.
Children (2-16 years old): adjust the adult dose downwards, depending on the age of the child – see Chapter 6.

Babies: 2ml of chamomile tea for each month of age (i.e. 0-1 month old – 2ml of tea; 2 months old – 4ml of tea; etc), 1-3 times a day.

OPTIONAL HERBS

HOPS

> **Warning:** Avoid if you have oestrogen-sensitive breast cancer or a tendency towards depression.

Uses
Hops make a strong relaxant and help with sleep problems. They are suitable for people who are anxious, who worry too much or who cannot drop off to sleep.

Combinations
Hops combine well with valerian and passion-flower for insomnia.

How to take
As tincture.

Dosage
Adults: 0.5-1ml diluted with some water, 1-3 times a day, tincture strength 1:2.
Children (2-16 years old): adjust the adult dose downwards, depending on the age of the child – see Chapter 6.

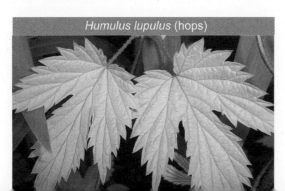
Humulus lupulus (hops)

LEMON BALM

Uses
Lemon balm is somewhat similar to lime tree flower: it gently relaxes and lifts the spirits, its actions being readily observable within half an hour of taking it. This herb is also very good for indigestion resulting from stress or anxiety. Drinking lemon balm tea before going to bed should ensure deep, uninterrupted sleep.

How to take
As tea. Try to make the tea from fresh leaves, as the taste and action of these is superior to that of the dry herb.

Dosage
Adults: 1-3 cups a day.
Children (2-16 years old): adjust the adult dose downwards, depending on the age of the child – see Chapter 6.

LIME TREE FLOWER

Uses
The tea made from lime tree flower has a relaxing effect on an anxious, overactive mind. It is traditionally drunk in parts of France as an after-dinner drink, because it will benefit your digestion as well as your sleep. Such tea lifts the spirits gently, in situations where stress has brought you down. It is also one of the nicest herbal teas to drink as it has a lovely aroma and pleasant taste, which can be enhanced with a little bit of honey. I regard this tea as the best remedy against the winter blues (it will warm you up as well!) or for when you feel down after having had a cold.

How to take

Dried flowers are normally used to make the tea. It is best drunk in the afternoon or evening to ensure sound sleep.

Dosage

Adults: 1-3 cups a day.

Children (2-16 years old): adjust the adult dose downwards, depending on the age of the child – see Chapter 6.

LIQUORICE

Warning: Do not take if you have high blood pressure; low potassium; heart, kidney or liver problems; or suffer from water retention. **Caution needed** if pregnant or elderly.

Uses

Liquorice affects the nervous system indirectly by supporting the function of the adrenal glands. The adrenal glands are responsible for the swift responses of the nervous system in stressful situations, and can become exhausted if you are continually stressed. Liquorice gently supports the adrenals, which has a positive effect on mood and emotions. I recommend this herb at times of prolonged stress and for emotional fragility, mild depression and general nervous exhaustion.

How to take

For all these purposes a strong tincture is the best form. If you have a tendency towards water retention or high blood pressure, take only half of the recommended dose for a week at a time, then have a week's break. You can repeat this on-off procedure for 2-3 months.

Dosage

Adults: 0.4-1.6ml diluted with some water, 1-3 times a day, tincture strength 1:1.

Children (2-16 years old): adjust the adult dose downwards, depending on the age of the child – see Chapter 6.

OATS

Uses

Oats have a special place among the herbs used to help the nervous system – they are the restorative herb for this system. I recommend resorting to oats when you feel mentally or emotionally exhausted, when you have lost your motivation and drive, or generally when you have been under a lot of stress for a prolonged period of time. Oats support the nervous system and heal it after it has been under continual strain.

Combinations

Oats can be mixed with any herbs that are relaxing, anti-anxiety or antidepressant.

How to take

As tincture, which should be made from fresh green oats or oat straw.

Dosage

Adults: 1-2ml diluted with some water, 2-3 times a day, tincture strength 1:2.

Children (2-16 years old): adjust the adult dose downwards, depending on the age of the child – see Chapter 6.

PASSIONFLOWER

Uses
Passionflower is primarily a remedy for insomnia and anxiety. It is a good substitute for valerian in cases of sleep problems, but it is more suitable for long-term anxiety rather than, say, stage fright or exam nerves.

Combinations
It combines well with hops, lemon balm and valerian for the treatment of long-term anxiety.

Dosage
Adults: 0.5-2ml diluted with some water, 1-3 times a day, tincture strength 1:2.
Children (2-16 years old): adjust the adult dose downwards, depending on the age of the child – see Chapter 6.

ROSE

Uses
Very few people realise that rose is an anti-depressant. This herb is used in the Middle East as a remedy for shock and bereavement. Women seem to respond better to this herb than men, and I recommend using it for depressive moods related to hormonal fluctuations, including the menopausal ones.

How to use
Use it as tincture, made from fresh petals. Good-quality rose tincture is not easy to buy so you may have to make your own. You need to use red or pink roses with a strong fragrance, preferably *Rosa damascena*, *Rosa centifolia* or *Rosa gallica*. You can also use rose essential oil (called otto) in a vaporiser or in your bath to lift the spirits (general precautions for essential oils apply – see page 23).

Combinations
Rose combines well with lemon balm, St John's wort and vervain.

Dosage
Adults: 1-2ml diluted with some water, 2-3 times a day, tincture strength 1:2.
Children (2-16 years old): adjust the adult dose downwards, depending on the age of the child – see Chapter 6.

ST JOHN'S WORT

Caution: Seek specialist advice if on any medication. Avoid excessive exposure to sun or UV light. These cautions do not apply to the infused oil of St John's wort.

Uses
This herb is familiar to many people as a natural antidepressant. It works well for mild-to-moderate depression. St John's wort can be used in any circumstances where low mood is a symptom, but it is especially helpful for menopausal mood swings and post-viral depression. St John's wort is non-addictive, unlike many conventional antidepressants and has mild anti-anxiety properties. It is also a restorative herb for the nervous tissue, which means that it helps the recovery from illnesses of the nervous tissue (e.g. neuralgia) or injury to this tissue.

The quality of preparation is the key to this herb's effectiveness, so it is worth investing in high-quality products (see Resources section). St John's wort works relatively quickly in my experience – within a week or two – but occasionally people need to persevere for longer to feel the uplifting effect. If you don't experience a significant improvement within six weeks you should seek an alternative treatment.

Combinations

St John's wort combines well with rose, vervain and valerian, the latter in situations where anxiety is a pronounced feature.

How to take

Tincture is preferable to tea.

You should not take St John's wort if you are on any medication without consulting a medical herbalist – this herb can alter the effectiveness of many drugs, even the Pill. In most cases it is a matter of setting the appropriate dose that is compatible with conventional types of medication. I do not recommend tinctures standardised to one constituent because the effectiveness of this herb depends on the whole spectrum of many constituents, not just a single one.

Dosage

Adults: 0.6-2ml diluted with some water, 2-3 times a day, tincture strength 1:2.
Children (2-16 years old): adjust the adult dose downwards, depending on the age of the child – see Chapter 6.

VERVAIN

Uses

Vervain is a gentle relaxant and antidepressant. One of its actions is helping the body to cope with stress or recover from the effects of stress. Vervain can be used in situations where prolonged stress begins to show in the form of exhaustion, irritation or a low mood. It is also very helpful in recovering from illnesses that leave you depressed and unenergetic,

especially if your digestion is not functioning properly. A low mood and emotional swings that accompany menopausal changes also improve with vervain.

How to take

As a tincture or tea.

Dosage

Adults: 1-2ml diluted with some water, 1-3 times a day, tincture strength 1:2; or 1-3 cups of vervain tea a day.
Children (2-16 years old): adjust the adult dose downwards, depending on the age of the child – see Chapter 6.

SPECIFIC AILMENTS OF THE NERVOUS SYSTEM AND HERBS THAT CAN HELP

ANXIETY

Anxiety can be brought on by many circumstances and you may need professional help to overcome a persistent or severe form. Occasional anxiety relating to common life events such as a job interview, travelling, moving house, giving a presentation, etc. can be helped by taking relaxing herbs. All these herbs work relatively quickly – within half an hour of taking them.

Treatment options

- Take valerian tincture. *Adults (for regular use for up to a month):* 0.3-1ml diluted with some water, 1-3 times a day, tincture strength 1:1.
Adults (for one-off use): 5ml diluted with

some water 2 hours before a stressful event; another 5ml diluted with some water half an hour before.

- Drink chamomile tea on a regular basis (for precautions see page 82). *Adults:* 2-3 cups a day; use 2 teaspoonsful of loose herbs per cup or two tea bags.

- Take passionflower tincture if anxiety stops you from sleeping. *Adults:* 0.5-2ml diluted with some water, 1-3 times a day, tincture strength 1:2.

- Drink lemon balm tea. *Adults:* 1-3 cups a day.

- Take the anti-anxiety mix (see box, right).

Children (2-16 years old): adjust the adult dose downwards, depending on the age of the child – see Chapter 6.

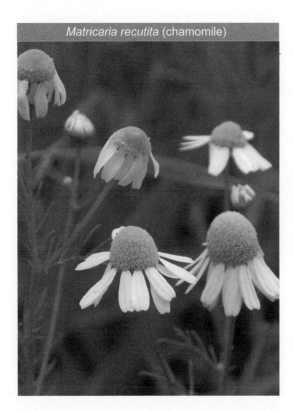
Matricaria recutita (chamomile)

ANTI-ANXIETY MIX

Ingredients
- 20ml hops (tincture strength 1:2) (for precautions see page 83)
- 20ml lemon balm (tincture strength 1:2)
- 30ml valerian (tincture strength 1:1)
- 30ml passionflower (tincture strength 1:2)

To make
- Mix ingredients together.
- Pour into a clean, dark glass bottle.
- Label with the contents and the date.
- Store at room temperature for up to a year.

Adult dose: 5ml diluted with some water, 2-3 times a day.

CONCENTRATION, LACK OF

Lack of concentration can be improved with diet, supplements, herbs and adjustments to lifestyle. Herbs will rarely provide the whole answer if there is a long-standing problem. The measures below are useful for situations when you need to concentrate for extra-long periods of time: for instance, when studying for an exam or driving a long distance. Often poor concentration results from lack of sleep, so relaxing herbs taken before going to bed will improve your concentration the next day.

Treatment options
- Take Siberian ginseng tincture (for precautions see page 152). *Adults:* 1-4ml, 1-2 times a day, tincture strength 1:2.

- Use rosemary essential oil (for precautions see page 82). *Adults:* add 5 drops to a bath;

or use 2-3 drops in a vaporiser; or crush a twig of fresh rosemary in your fingers and inhale the fragrance for a few seconds and repeat whenever your concentration begins to flag again.

Children (2-16 years old): adjust the adult dose downwards, depending on the age of the child – see Chapter 6.

Depression

Practitioner treatment is recommended for this condition.

A low mood can be lifted with many herbs, but severe depression needs help from a health professional. If you try the measures below, either singly or in combination, and you do not get results within six weeks, seek advice from a herbalist or your GP. Depression is a complex disease and often herbs other than antidepressant ones are required. For instance, if your depression is related to your periods you may need herbs to balance your hormones, or if you feel down after having flu you will need herbs that boost your immune system.

Treatment options

- Take St John's wort tincture (for precautions see page 85). *Adults:* 0.6-2ml diluted with some water, 2-3 times a day, tincture strength 1:2.

- Take rose tincture. *Adults:* 1-2ml diluted with some water, 2-3 times a day, tincture strength 1:2.

- Take vervain tincture or tea. *Adults:* 1-2ml diluted with some water, 1-3 times a day,

tincture strength 1:2; or 1-3 cups of vervain tea a day.

- Take oats tincture. *Adults:* 1-2ml diluted with some water, 2-3 times a day, tincture strength 1:2.

- Use rosemary essential oil (for precautions see page 82). *Adults:* 5 drops added to a bath; or 2-3 drops in a vaporiser.

- If anxiety is one of your symptoms, take the mix for mild depression with anxiety – see box below.

MIX FOR MILD DEPRESSION WITH ANXIETY

Ingredients
- 20ml rose (tincture strength 1:2)
- 30ml vervain (tincture strength 1:2)
- 20ml valerian (tincture strength 1:1)
- 30ml St John's wort (tincture strength 1:2) (for precautions see page 85)

To make
- Mix ingredients together.
- Pour into a clean, dark glass bottle.
- Label with the contents and the date.

Adult dose: 5ml diluted with some water, 2-3 times a day.

Children (2-16 years old): adjust the adult dose downwards, depending on the age of the child – see Chapter 6.

Exam nerves / stage fright

Most of us get nervous before big events such as sitting an exam or speaking in public. Herbs can take the edge of such nervousness, yet will not diminish your performance. Depending on how nervous you get, you can opt for milder herbs, for example lemon balm, or stronger-acting ones such as valerian or passionflower, and you can vary the dosage according to your need. All the herbs below are suitable for children who get nervous before taking exams.

Treatment options

- Take valerian tincture. *Adults:* take 5ml diluted with some water, tincture strength 1:1, a few hours before the event, and then another 5ml diluted with some water half an hour before the event. If the event is in the evening you may need a dose in the morning, one at lunchtime and then another half an hour before the event. Do not be tempted to take a double dose in one go as that can send you to sleep!

- Take passionflower tincture. *Adults:* 0.5-2ml diluted with some water, 1-3 times a day, tincture strength 1:2.

- Drink lemon balm tea. *Adults:* 1-3 cups a day.

Children (2-16 years old): adjust the adult dose downwards, depending on the age of the child – see Chapter 6.

HEADACHE (TENSION)

A headache can have many causes, for instance dehydration, tension or eye strain. The most common type is tension headache, which is related mainly to stress and sometimes to problems with the neck vertebrae. If you suffer from headaches a lot, it may be worth seeing a herbalist for an individual prescription that will address the root cause of your headaches and also contain painkiller herbs not available over the counter.

Treatment options

- Take valerian tincture. *Adults:* 5ml, 1-2 times a day, tincture strength 1:1, if you already have a headache; or 0.3-1ml, 1-3 times a day, for a few weeks to prevent tension headaches if you get a lot of them.

- Drink lavender tea. *Adults:* 1 cup as soon as you feel the headache coming on; use 1 teaspoonful of loose herbs per cup.

- Drink lemon balm tea. *Adults:* 1-2 cups when you feel the headache coming on.

- Drink chamomile tea (for precautions see page 82). *Adults:* 1-2 cups when you feel the headache coming on.

- Drink the tea for tension headaches – see box.

> **TEA FOR TENSION HEADACHES**
> Ingredients
> - 25g dry lavender
> - 25g dry lemon balm
> - 25g dry chamomile (for precautions see page 82)
> - 25g dry lime tree flower
>
> To make
> - Mix herbs thoroughly.
> - Infuse 2 teaspoonsful of the mix in a cupful of freshly boiled water for 10 minutes. Strain and drink warm. You can add honey to this tea.
>
> Adult dose: 1-2 cups when you feel the headache coming on.

- Drink lime tree flower tea. *Adults:* 1-2 cups when you feel the headache coming on.

Children (2-16 years old): adjust the adult dose downwards, depending on the age of the child – see Chapter 6.

INSOMNIA

Practitioner treatment is recommended for this condition.

Insomnia can be successfully treated with sleep-inducing herbs and there is no danger of becoming addicted to such herbs. Often, when you are under a lot of stress, you need both a daytime treatment to help you relax and a night-time treatment to help you drop off to sleep. The options below are meant mostly for one-off situations when you find it difficult to fall asleep or expect to have difficulty falling asleep.

Treatment options

• Take valerian tincture; it is very good in situations when your mind is still very active in spite of the late hour. *Adults:* 5ml diluted with some water, tincture strength 1:1, once, if you cannot fall asleep. If you find yourself slightly groggy in the morning reduce the dose next time to 2-3ml.

• Put lavender essential oil in a bath or directly on the pillow you will sleep on (for

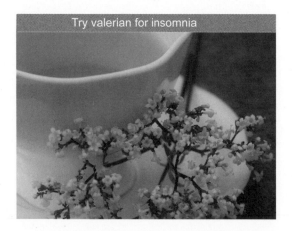
Try valerian for insomnia

precautions see page 81). *Adults:* 5 drops in a bath; 2-3 drops on a pillow.

• If you have had problems with sleeping for a long time, prepare a mix for insomnia (see box) and take it regularly for a month.

> **MIX FOR INSOMNIA**
> Ingredients
> • 40ml valerian (tincture strength 1:1)
> • 30ml hops (tincture strength 1:2) (for precautions see page 83)
> • 30ml passionflower (tincture strength 1:2)
>
> To make
> • Mix ingredients together.
> • Pour into a clean, dark glass bottle.
> • Label with the contents and the date.
> • Store at room temperature for up to a year.
>
> Adult dose: 5ml diluted with some water half an hour before sleep.

Children (2-16 years old): adjust the adult dose downwards, depending on the age of the child – see Chapter 6.

• Have a hops pillow or lavender pillow next to your head in bed so that you can smell and inhale the fragrance; you can make your own by buying about 100-200g of loose herbs and stuffing a small muslin bag with the herbs. Small lavender pillows are suitable for children.

• For children, chamomile tea before bed is usually sufficient to induce sleep. *Children:* 2-3 years old – ¼ cup; 4-8 years old – ½ cup; 8-12 years old – full cup.

NERVOUS INDIGESTION

Indigestion is often the result of anxiety or worry. At such times, the measures below can be used singly or together, depending on how severe the symptoms are; all the measures can be used long-term (6-12 months) if necessary.

Treatment options

- Drink chamomile tea freely (for precautions see page 82). *Adults:* 3-4 cups a day; if you suffer from heartburn limit this to 1 cup a day.

- Supplement the above with valerian tincture. *Adults:* 1-2ml diluted with some water, 1-2 times a day, tincture strength 1:1.

- Take marshmallow root powder if you get heartburn due to stress (for precautions see page 48).

Children (2-16 years old): adjust the adult dose downwards, depending on the age of the child – see Chapter 6.

NEURALGIA

Neuralgia is a pain caused by damage to or inflammation of the nervous tissue. The most common types of neuralgia are: trigeminal neuralgia, neuralgia that can follow shingles or herpes, and neuralgia associated with sciatica. Irrespective of which type, you will benefit from both internal treatment and the external application of herbs that are anti-inflammatory and regenerative to the nervous tissue. The antiviral properties of St John's wort come in useful for neuralgia associated with shingles or herpes; use internally as a tincture and externally as an infused oil.

Treatment options

- Take St John's wort tincture; you will need maximum doses until the pain subsides, then reduce to the middle range of the dose until the pain disappears. For precautions see page 85. *Adults:* 2ml diluted with some water, 3 times a day, tincture strength 1:2; then reducing to 1ml diluted with some water, 3 times a day.

- Take passionflower tincture for its calming and painkilling properties. *Adults:* 0.5-2ml, 3 times a day, tincture strength 1:2.

- Take hops tincture to reduce nerve hyper-sensitivity (for precautions see page 83). *Adults:* 0.5-1ml, 2-3 times a day, tincture strength 1:2.

Children (2-16 years old): adjust the adult dose downwards, depending on the age of the child – see Chapter 6.

- Apply St John's wort infused oil externally over the affected area. *Adults and children:* apply the oil 2-4 times a day.

PANIC ATTACKS

Practitioner treatment is recommended for this condition.

Occasional panic attacks can be overcome with the measures given below. Breathing into a paper bag during an attack is an effective measure for bringing the breath rate back to normal. In general, however, panic attacks are indicative of extreme anxiety, in which case professional help would be more effective as herbalists can prescribe an individual prescription with strong sedative properties.

Treatment options

- Take valerian tincture. *Adults:* 10ml, once, diluted with some water, tincture strength 1:1, during a panic attack; or 5-10ml a day as a preventative measure.

- Drink strong lemon balm tea as a preventative measure. *Adults:* 2-3 cups a day.

Children (2-16 years old): adjust the adult dose downwards, depending on the age of the child – see Chapter 6.

SHINGLES

Practitioner treatment is recommended for this condition.

Shingles is a chicken pox virus 'resurfacing', usually when one's immune system is not working as well as it should. The treatment below, both internal and external, should bring quick relief. If you are not getting satisfactory results, consult a herbalist for stronger immune support and antiviral herbs.

Treatment options

- Take echinacea tincture (for precautions see page 98). *Adults:* 1-2ml, 3 times a day, tincture strength 1:5. *Children (2-16 years old):* adjust the adult dose downwards, depending on the age of the child – see Chapter 6.

- Apply the ointment for shingles described above right – it will ease the pain and speed up the recovery (precautions for essential oils apply).

OINTMENT FOR SHINGLES

Ingredients

- 50g calendula ointment or cream (for precautions see page 114)
- 20 drops lemon balm essential oil (for precautions see page 53)

To make

- Mix well.
- Transfer to a clean, dark glass jar, making sure that there are no air pockets left.
- Store for up to 12 months.

Adults and children over 3 years old: apply to the affected area twice a day.

STRESS

Coping with stress is not always easy, and our ability to manage it varies throughout our lives and according to the nature of the stress. Siberian ginseng can increase your resistance to stress: it works as a general tonic for all body systems including the nervous system, and it makes you more resilient to life's pressures. I recommend using Siberian ginseng in specific situations when you expect an unusual increase in stress: for instance, during exams or when you need to meet deadlines at work. Korean ginseng works in a similar way, but it is much stronger and is considered not suitable for anyone under 40. The ability to cope with stress can be also related to your adrenal function, which can be improved with specific herbs but is best treated under the supervision of a herbalist. See also Chapter 18.

Treatment options

- Take Siberian ginseng tincture to increase your resistance to stress – this herb can be taken long term; for many months if necessary. For precautions see page 152. *Adults:* 1-4ml diluted with some water, 1-2 times a day, tincture strength 1:2.

- Take valerian tincture if your reaction to stress manifests itself as anxiety or irritability. *Adults:* 0.3-1ml diluted with some water, 1-3 times a day, tincture strength 1:1.

- Take liquorice tincture if prolonged stress has left you exhausted (for precautions see page 84). *Adults:* 0.4-1.6ml diluted with some water, 1-3 times a day, tincture strength 1:1.

- Take oats tincture if prolonged stress has left you exhausted and depressed. *Adults:* 1-2ml diluted with some water, 2-3 times a day, tincture strength 1:2.

Children (2-16 years old): adjust the adult dose downwards, depending on the age of the child – see Chapter 6.

WHEN AND WHY YOU SHOULD SEE A PROFESSIONAL MEDICAL HERBALIST

- Migraine: this condition has many causes, often related to dietary factors or hormonal imbalances.

- Depression that does not respond quickly to St John's wort: there are many herbs that can lift mood but they need to be matched to the individual.

- Pronounced anxiety: this problem requires careful adjustment of specific herbs and their dosage.

- Neuralgia: this ailment requires a careful balance of herbal painkillers with the herbs that restore the nervous tissue back to health.

- Multiple sclerosis: this is a disease affecting nerve tissue that can, in the early stages, be successfully put in remission by individualised herbal treatment. In cases of advanced disease herbs can offer much in terms of supportive treatment.

- Shingles: this condition responds very well to herbal treatment but may require specific immune stimulation.

THE FOLLOWING SYMPTOMS WARRANT SEEING A HEALTH PROFESSIONAL WITHOUT DELAY

- Prolonged or very severe headache.

- A sudden change to your vision or hearing.

- Unusual sensations in your limbs (pins and needles, numbness).

- Extreme anxiety.

- Severe depression.

Chapter 14
The respiratory system

This chapter deals with problems associated with the respiratory system. The main parts of the respiratory system are the nose, throat and lungs. The ears and sinuses are closely associated with the respiratory system and are therefore included here as well. This system tends to be diseased more often than other systems as it is very easy to pick up all sorts of bugs by just breathing them in. Common infections of the respiratory system are usually viral but can occasionally be bacterial in origin. It is useful to distinguish between the two to choose the best treatment, herbal or conventional. The differences are pointed out in this chapter when discussing specific ailments in detail. Sometimes it is not possible to say whether you have been infected by a virus or bacteria unless you have a specialist investigation.

TEMPERATURE

An important point to remember with infections of the respiratory system is that there is a direct link between body temperature and the severity of the infection: the higher the temperature, the 'nastier' the bug. Children are more likely to run a high fever very quickly, so it is really important to check on it often and keep it down with appropriate measures (see the section on fever, page 108).

NUTRITION

Before moving on to herbal treatment I would like to advocate a couple of nutritional measures that are useful aids when treating the common cold.

The first one is the traditional advice to drink lemon juice and honey with hot water. It makes good sense as honey has mild antibiotic properties, soothes the lining of the throat, boosts your energy and warms you up, while lemon juice provides vitamin C, which reduces catarrh. You can use manuka honey for extra antibiotic properties – manuka honey is made by bees using pollen from the flowering tea tree plant. Use hot water but let it cool a bit after boiling as very hot water will destroy vitamin C in lemon juice. I usually mix 2 teaspoonsful of honey with 1 teaspoon of lemon juice per cup of water, but you can use your own proportions according to taste.

The second traditional food that helps with colds or flu-like symptoms is chicken broth, which is a common treatment in many European countries. This has been confirmed by a number of researchers.[3] In the box opposite is a recipe that I use at home; I recommend that you cook your own – it will have more nutrients than a tinned or packet version.

You want to have clear broth, so do not blend the ingredients. I normally add some precooked noodles or rice to the broth, plus chunks of carrots and chicken meat. It is the most comforting, fortifying meal if you have a cold, but is also good when convalescing from any serious illness. I have not come across a good vegetarian equivalent, so my apologies to vegetarian readers; however miso soup is close in terms of taste and mineral content.

RECIPE FOR CHICKEN BROTH

Ingredients
- 4 drumsticks or 2 thighs –choose any parts of the chicken, preferably organic, with bones and skin
- 5 whole peeled carrots
- 2 parsnips
- 1 onion
- 1 litre water

To make
- Cover chicken with water.
- Boil for about ½ hour.
- Add carrots, parsnips and onion.
- Keep boiling on a low setting until the vegetables are tender.
- Add salt and pepper to taste.

REST

Finally, there has been a marked increase in people suffering from post-viral fatigue over the last few years. This is not coincidental but largely a consequence of the fact that we are expected to push ourselves when we have a cold, instead of staying in bed and then at home until we recover. Two to five days at home will give your body enough time to recuperate properly and also to stop spreading the infection to other people. Please refer to the section on recovering from serious illness (Chapter 22) if you have had flu, glandular fever, bronchitis or a nasty cold that you can't shake off.

MUST-HAVE HERBS

The herbs in this section are listed in order of usefulness.

ELDERFLOWER

This is my favourite herb for helping both to prevent the development of a cold or flu and for lessening the symptoms. Elderflower tea is the most effective treatment against viral infections in my view.

Uses
Elderflower can be used both for nipping a cold in the bud and for the treatment of various symptoms of a cold. Ideally, if you start taking it right at the onset of symptoms you should not develop a cold at all, but if you do, it is still worth taking elderflower tea or tincture as you will recover more quickly and your symptoms will be milder. Apart from being antiviral, elderflower has anti-catarrhal properties, so it is especially worth taking this tea or tincture in situations when catarrh is a prominent symptom, and this applies to an ordinary runny nose as well as to allergic reactions and hay fever. As elderflower is a warming herb you can feel quite hot for a short while after taking it, especially after drinking a hot elderflower tea. This warming effect is useful for reducing a mildly raised temperature.

Elderflower tea is noticeably diuretic, so make sure you drink plenty of water to compensate and avoid drinking it just before going to bed, unless you do not mind getting up in the middle of the night.

Commercially made elderflower cordials do not have any appreciable medicinal properties.

Combinations
Elderflower combines well with garlic in any form.

How to take
Elderflower needs to be taken at the earliest possible stage of a cold or flu-like illness if you want to prevent it. You need between 2 and 4 cups of infusion a day to prevent a cold from developing. It is most common to drink 4 cups on the day you start feeling under the weather and 1-2 cups on the following day. Each cup should be brewed with 2 teaspoonsful of dry herbs per cup or 2-4 tablespoons of fresh flowers. It is best to make a fresh brew of tea each time and drink it warm. You can add honey to it if you wish.

In my experience, warm, freshly brewed elderflower tea works best of all the possible preparations that can be made from elderflower, but the tincture is also quite effective and may appeal to people who are travelling and who dislike the elderflower tea taste.

Dosage
Adults: 1 cup of infusion 1-4 times a day; or 5-15ml, 2-3 times a day, tincture strength 1:5. *Children (2-16 years old):* adjust the adult dose downwards, depending on the age of the child – see Chapter 6.

GARLIC

Warning: Do not take large doses for prolonged periods of time or when pregnant or breastfeeding. Not suitable for children under 6 years old.
Caution needed if taking anti-coagulant or anti-platelet medication.

Uses
Garlic is a superb anti-cold agent. You can take it in capsule form, eat it raw or drink garlic juice. Taking garlic regularly through the winter will prevent many milder colds, or you can take it in larger doses to treat a cold that is already under way. However, garlic can be too strong for very small children and is not always compatible with other medication: for instance, large amounts should not be taken with any blood-thinning medication such as warfarin. When garlic is cooked it loses most of its medicinal properties and it is safe to be consumed in all circumstances.

It is important that you choose a good-quality preparation: look for freeze-dried garlic capsules/tablets that list the allicin or alliin content. This is the most active ingredient of garlic, which is also responsible for its smell.

Combinations
Garlic combines well with elderflower for the treatment of colds.

How to take
You can make your own garlic juice, if you have a juicer, and freeze it into small cubes, about a teaspoonful each, and then use it when you need it, mixed with water or fruit juice as you would do with tinctures. Mixing garlic juice with fruit juice sounds odd but tastes fine, especially if it is mango juice. Alternatively, you can stabilise the juice with alcohol for long-term storage (see box opposite).

From my personal observation, confirmed by all my patients who have used garlic juice, I have found that it does not give you garlicky breath! You will experience an aftertaste for a short while but it does not linger, and if you mix garlic juice with any fruit juice you will hardly notice it at all.

However, the simplest way of taking garlic is to chop a single clove very finely, or crush it in a garlic press, mix it with a generous spoonful of honey and just swallow the lot. You can drink some water or juice to help it go down. The honey will mask the taste of garlic quite effectively, yet preserve garlic's curative, antimicrobial properties.

I do not advocate taking raw garlic all the time in large amounts (3 cloves a day counts as a large dose), as such a habit may alter the bowel flora and lead to digestive problems; the same applies to garlic capsules and juice. Of course, cooked garlic is an entirely different matter, and you can have it all the time without any harmful effect.

Dosage

Adults: 1 teaspoon of garlic juice, either freshly squeezed, defrosted or stabilised with alcohol, 1-3 times a day; or a crushed clove, 1-3 times a day, mixed with honey. If you opt for garlic capsules/tablets, follow the manufacturer's instructions for use.

Children (6-16 years old): adjust the adult dose downwards, depending on the age of the child – see Chapter 6.

LONG-LIFE GARLIC JUICE
Ingredients
- 150ml freshly squeezed garlic juice (use a juicer). For precautions see page 96
- 250ml of 40% pure vodka or brandy

To make
- Mix the juice and alcohol together.
- Pour into a clean, dark glass bottle.
- Label with the contents and the date.
- Store for up to 2 years in a cool, dark, place.

ONION

Uses

Onion is milder than garlic but particularly effective for chest infections and most types of cough. Fresh onion has an antimicrobial effect in the airways, as well as being soothing. Onion will reduce the intensity and frequency of coughing, and your cough should go away quite quickly. Being a common food item that happens to have curative properties, it is safe in all circumstances and for all age groups.

How to take

I recommend using freshly made onion syrup, which will work best when taken as soon as you develop a cough. I got the recipe given overleaf from one of my teachers when I was training as a herbalist, and after the very first time of using it I became its firm advocate. Although the idea of onion syrup may not be tremendously appealing when it first springs to mind, it tastes surprisingly nice, if you ignore the smell of raw onion . . . It is also easy to make when travelling –I made it once when trekking in the Himalayas. You can take onion syrup by itself or with any other herbal syrup.

Dosage

Adults: 1 teaspoonful, 4-5 times a day until symptoms improve; for a slight cough take 1 teaspoonful 1-2 times a day; or for a severe cough take 1 teaspoonful 7-8 times a day.

Children (2-16 years old): adjust the adult dose downwards, depending on the age of the child – see Chapter 6.

RECIPE FOR ONION SYRUP

Ingredients
- 1 large onion
- 5-7 teaspoonsful of brown sugar or honey

To make
- Peel and slice the onion into chunky slices about 5mm thick.
- Put one slice in a cup and cover with a spoonful of sugar or honey.
- Follow with layers of onion slices and sugar/honey.
- Leave the cup covered for a few hours.
- The sugar will extract the juice from the onion and you can collect the resulting syrup in a different cup (keep it covered for storage) or a small bottle.
- Do not store for longer than 2 days.

Note: This syrup works only when freshly made, so you may have to make a fresh batch every 2 days if necessary. One onion produces on average 2 days' worth of syrup.

ECHINACEA (PURPLE CONEFLOWER)

Caution needed if allergic to plants of the *Compositae* family.

Uses

The latest research[4] on the use of echinacea species and prevention of colds favours continuous use through the autumn and winter. This approach prepares the immune system to respond more quickly to viral infections and in effect you do not develop any symptoms or, if you catch a cold, the symptoms are much milder. There are two distinct species that are used medicinally: *Echinacea purpurea* and *Echinacea pallida* var. *angustifolia* (often referred to as *E. angustifolia*). A combination of *Echinacea angustifolia* and *Echinacea purpurea* **roots** works best and I would recommend that you buy it from bona fide herbalists to ensure good quality. *Echinacea angustifolia* is virtually extinct in the wild through over-harvesting, so be sure to buy only from the cultivated sources – it will be expensive because it is difficult to grow. *Echinacea purpurea* is, however, easily cultivated in this country and, although less medicinally effective, is a better environmental choice. There is a simple test to assess the quality of echinacea tincture: if you put a drop or two of the neat tincture on your tongue you should feel a strong tingling sensation that is caused by alkylamides, the most relevant active constituents of the plant. If you feel no tingling, you have wasted your money.

How to take

I generally prescribe this herb in tincture form and long-term for people whose immune system is weakened – they catch all the bugs that are going round – or for those who take ages to recover from a particular infection. As a rule, I would avoid taking echinacea if you have severe symptoms as it can occasionally make them worse.

I have found elderflower tea to be more effective in nipping a cold in the bud than echinacea, and it is certainly a cheaper option. However, I know plenty of people who use echinacea in larger doses at the onset of symptoms and get good results (a large dose is 5ml 3 times a day of 1:5 tincture, while a long-term-use adult dose is 1-2ml 3 times a day of 1:5 tincture). By careful experimenting you can find out what works best for you.

People who are prone to allergies should exercise caution with echinacea, as it is known to cause occasional allergic reaction, usually in the form of a skin rash. Start with very small doses if you have never taken it before, especially if you suffer from asthma, eczema or hay fever. Certain inflammatory disorders, for instance, rheumatoid arthritis, can be worsened occasionally by taking echinacea.

Dosage

Adults: for long-term use take 1-2ml diluted with some water, 3 times a day, tincture strength 1:5; or for short, intense treatment take 5ml diluted with some water 3 times a day, tincture strength 1:5.

Children (2-16 years old): adjust the adult dose downwards, depending on the age of the child – see Chapter 6.

PROPOLIS

> **Warning:** Not suitable for children under 3 years old.
>
> **Caution needed** if you have a history of allergy.

Uses

Propolis is a bee product and comes from a variety of tree resins. Bees make propolis to protect the hive from any infections, and it is a powerful natural 'antibiotic' with a large spectrum of action against a wide range of bacteria, viruses and fungi. Propolis can be used for a variety of respiratory system problems: sore throat, tonsillitis, flu, chest infections, bad coughs, nasty colds or bronchitis.

Propolis has been shown to enhance the action of many antibiotics when taken at the same time.

Combinations

Propolis combines well with elderflower and echinacea in any form.

How to take

You can use propolis spray (made from propolis tincture 1:10) or propolis lozenges for sore throats, irrespective of whether the infection is viral or bacterial. By spraying the liquid directly to the back of the throat you will be delivering a powerful local treatment, although the taste of propolis tincture is quite strong and you may experience some stinging. You should use the spray as soon as you develop a sore throat. Otherwise you can take propolis internally, either as tincture or capsules. Buy only from reputable suppliers as quality can be an issue.

Dosage

Adults: 1-2ml diluted with some water, 1-3 times a day, tincture strength 1:10; or 1g of powdered propolis in capsule or tablet form, 1-3 times a day; or 1-2 puffs from a spray bottle to the back of the throat, 2-4 times a day; or propolis lozenges – take according to the manufacturer's instructions.

Children (3-16 years old): adjust the adult dose downwards, depending on the age of the child – see Chapter 6.

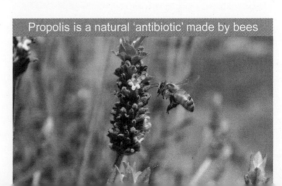
Propolis is a natural 'antibiotic' made by bees

THYME

Uses
Thyme is a powerful antiseptic for the lungs and therefore useful for chesty colds with a bad cough, especially a dry one.

Combinations
Thyme combines well in tincture form with liquorice, elecampane and ground ivy for the treatment of chest infections, especially if the cough lingers on for weeks.

How to take
Thyme is best taken as tincture or as a thyme and liquorice syrup (for precautions see page 101).

Refer to Chapter 26 if you want to make your own thyme and liquorice syrup, otherwise you can purchase it directly from practising herbalists who run their own apothecaries.

Dosage
Adults: 0.7-1.5ml diluted with some water, 1-3 times a day, tincture strength 1:2; or thyme and liquorice syrup, 1 teaspoonful 2-5 times a day.
Children (2-16` years old): adjust the adult dose downwards, depending on the age of the child – see Chapter 6.

OPTIONAL HERBS

There are many herbs that can lower the temperature, take away the chill and soothe muscular aches and pains. You can customise your treatment according to your symptoms. For instance, if you have a cough, add one or two herbs that are specific for coughs. Some of these may be growing in your garden, in which case it makes sense to use what you already have.

ELECAMPANE

Uses
Elecampane root is a traditional remedy for chest infections. It has a disinfecting action on the lung tissue as well as being an expectorant. It can be used for any type of cough of recent origin, or to get rid of a lingering one.

Combinations
Elecampane works well in combination with ground ivy, liquorice and thyme or elderflower (see the mix on page 107).

How to take
As tincture.

Dosage
Adults: 1-2ml diluted with some water, 2-3 times a day, tincture strength 1:2.
Children (2-16 years old): adjust the adult dose downwards, depending on the age of the child – see Chapter 6.

GROUND IVY

Uses
Ground ivy belongs to the group of herbs that helps restore specific tissues to their healthy state. Ground ivy has a reputation for healing the lining of the respiratory tract. It provides a supportive treatment for coughs that drag on and cannot be shaken off.

Combinations
Ground ivy mixes well with the tinctures of elecampane, thyme and marshmallow root or liquorice root to treat lingering chest infections (see page 107).

How to take

Ground ivy is best used as tincture in combination with antimicrobial herbs.

Dosage

Adults: 1-2ml diluted with some water, 2-3 times a day, tincture strength 1:2.
Children (2-16 years old): adjust the adult dose downwards, depending on the age of the child – see Chapter 6.

LIME TREE FLOWERS

Uses

Lime tree flowers are a traditional remedy used to reduce fever. This is a warming herb, which will induce slight perspiration if your body temperature is above normal. It will also help with restless sleep, which often troubles sick people.

Use it for a moderately high temperature (between 37°C/98.6°F and 38°C/100.4°F).

Combinations

You can combine it with elderflower.

How to take

Either as tea made from dry flowers or as tincture.

Dosage

Adults: 5-10ml diluted with some water, 1-3 times a day, tincture strength 1:5; or 1 cup of warm infusion, 1-3 times a day.
Children (2-16 years old): adjust the adult dose downwards, depending on the age of the child – see Chapter 6.

LIQUORICE

Warning: Do not take when pregnant or if elderly.

Do not take long-term if you have high blood pressure, low potassium, heart/kidney/liver problems or water retention.

Uses

Liquorice is a demulcent (anti-irritant) and anti-inflammatory herb. It will reduce the irritation in the airways caused by infection and coughing. **People for whom long-term use of liquorice is not advised can safely use it for a few days to treat a cough.**

Combinations

Liquorice combines well with thyme, the latter having an antibacterial action and the former soothing the bronchi and throat.

How to take

Syrup made with liquorice and thyme is very effective for chest infections and it is my preferred preparation. By itself you can take liquorice as tincture, or as a powder, which should be mixed with water to the consistency of runny custard.

Dosage

Adults: 0.4-1.6ml diluted with some water, 1-3 times a day, tincture strength 1:1; or 1g of liquorice powder, 2-3 times a day, mixed with water; or thyme and liquorice syrup, 1 teaspoonful 2-5 times a day.
Children (2-16 years old): adjust the adult dose downwards, depending on the age of the child – see Chapter 6.

Marshmallow root

Uses
Marshmallow root, used as marshmallow syrup, is recommended specifically for a dry cough as it soothes the irritated airways. It is also good for a tickly cough resulting from a dry throat, which in turn often occurs when the nose is blocked with catarrh.

How to take
As an adult you can take this syrup freely (a teaspoonful at a time) whenever you have a bout of coughing, or throughout the day to prevent your throat from drying.

You can use marshmallow root tincture instead, although in my experience the syrup works better.

Dosage
Adults: 1 teaspoonful of syrup, 3-8 times a day; or 1-2ml diluted with some water, 1-3 times a day, tincture strength 1:5.
Children (2-16 years old): adjust the adult dose downwards, depending on the age of the child – see Chapter 6.

Mountain grape

Warning: Do not use when pregnant or breastfeeding.

Uses
I use mountain grape tincture as a substitute for golden seal, the latter being endangered in the wild and difficult to cultivate. Mountain grape has a wide range of antibacterial activity and is therefore good for bacterial infections of the sinuses, throat and chest. It is also mildly anti-catarrhal.

Combinations
Mountain grape combines well with thyme, elecampane and marshmallow tinctures for throat and chest infections.

How to take
As tincture.

Dosage
Adults: 1-2.5ml diluted with some water, 1-3 times a day, tincture strength 1:2.
Children (2-16 years old): adjust the adult dose downwards, depending on the age of the child – see Chapter 6.

Sage

Warning: Not suitable for internal treatment when pregnant.

Uses
Sage tea makes a soothing gargle for an inflamed throat as it is very astringent. I do not recommend its use internally for a cold as it inhibits sweating, which is a natural mechanism for bringing a high body temperature down.

How to take
Because sage is an evergreen plant I use it straight from my garden to make the gargle tea (10-15 chopped leaves per cup of boiled water), but you can also use dried sage (1-2 teaspoonsful per cup). I do not advise using the tincture as a gargle because it will sting (if you dilute it too much it will not have any effect). Children usually find this remedy too bitter, but if they are willing to try, let them do just one gargle once or twice a day. **Sage can be used as a gargle in pregnancy.**

Dosage
Adults: One mouthful of gargle, 3 times in a row. Repeat the procedure 3-4 times a day. *Children (5-16 years old):* One mouthful of gargle, 2 times in a row. Repeat the procedure 1-2 times a day.

St John's wort

Uses
St John's wort has antiviral and anti-inflammatory properties that come in useful for an external treatment for earache caused by an infection.

How to use
You will need a specific preparation of St John's wort that is called St John's wort infused oil. You can buy it ready-made from specialist retailers or make your own (see Chapter 26). For directions of usage see the earache entry in the next section of this chapter. Precautions for the internal use of St John's wort do not apply to the St John's wort infused oil.

SPECIFIC AILMENTS OF THE RESPIRATORY SYSTEM & HERBS THAT CAN HELP

Blocked nose, runny nose, catarrh
I am a great believer in allowing an ordinary runny nose to run, unpleasant though it is. Trying to suppress this normal reaction of the lining of the nose just prolongs the problem and often shifts the infection to the throat or chest. However, if your nose is so blocked that you can't breathe, the options below will ease the symptoms.

Try to opt for tissues made of organic cotton; they are far less irritating than ordinary tissues. If your nostrils end up feeling sore from blowing your nose all the time, apply a little calendula or comfrey ointment (see Chapter 15, page 114).

Treatment options
- Drink elderflower tea – it will reduce the secretions to a bearable level but will not suppress them completely; this anti-catarrhal effect is often noticeable within minutes of drinking the tea. *Adults:* 2-4 cups a day. *Children (2-16 years old):* adjust the adult dose downwards, depending on the age of the child – see Chapter 6.

- Inhale the steam from peppermint and thyme **tea** under a towel for 5-10 minutes (shorter time for children). *Adults and children above 5 years old:* 1-2 times a day.

- Inhale the steam from 2-3 drops each of rosemary and thyme essential oils in hot water under a towel for 5-10 minutes (shorter time for children). *Adults and children over 3 years old:* 1-2 times a day.

- Take fresh garlic (for precautions see page 96). *Adults:* 1-3 cloves a day; or 1-3 teaspoons of garlic juice a day. *Children:* Adjust downwards – see Chapter 6; not suitable for children under 6 years old.

Bronchitis

Practitioner treatment is recommended for this condition.

Bronchitis means inflammation of the bronchi, which are large airway branches leading to the lungs. The main symptoms are: persistent cough, either dry or productive, and fever. Herbalists see coughing as a natural body defence mechanism, not to be suppressed. They will use herbs to make coughing easier and less irritating, and to reduce the overall period of coughing. If your cough is dry, the aim is to make it productive, which means slightly stimulating the production of mucus. Productive cough is more effective at removing the infectious organism from the airways and it is less irritating to the bronchi. Herbs do not cause excessive mucus production. If your cough is already productive, the aim is to change the consistency of mucus so that it can be easily cleared from the lungs.

The best overall treatment is onion syrup, but you may need other syrups as well. Herbal syrups are very pure – they contain only herbs and sugar or honey – and therefore they do not cause drowsiness. They work by reducing irritation in the airways as well as by having a mild disinfectant action. You may need to approach your local herbalist if you want to keep any of them in stock, or make your own.

Bronchitis may have to be treated with a professional prescription from a herbalist or antibiotics from your doctor if there is any danger of it progressing to pneumonia.

Treatment options

- Take onion syrup (see page 98) – the best overall treatment. *Adults:* 1-8 teaspoonsful a day.

- Take marshmallow syrup for a dry cough. *Adults:* 3-8 teaspoonsful a day.

- Take thyme and liquorice syrup – chesty cough (for precautions see page 101). *Adults:* 1 teaspoonful 2-5 times a day.

- Drink elderflower tea to reduce temperature and in cases of a lot of catarrh. *Adults:* 1-3 cups a day.

- Take propolis tincture (for precautions see page 99). *Adults:* 1-2ml diluted with some water, 1-3 times a day, tincture strength 1:10; or 1-2g a day as capsules.

Children (2-16 years old): adjust the adult dose downwards, depending on the age of the child – see Chapter 6.

Colds, frequent

If you get more than your fair share of colds every winter (more than two or three), and if they linger for more than just a few days, your immune system may not be functioning very well. Many factors can be at play: for instance, your diet may be lacking in vital vitamins or minerals, or you may be under a lot of stress.

Treatment options

- Take echinacea tincture for a few months (for precautions see page 98). *Adults:* 1-2ml diluted with some water, 3 times a day, tincture strength 1:5.

- Drink elderflower tea during winter months. *Adults:* 1 cup a day.

- Include raw garlic in your diet or take garlic capsules, according to the manufacturer's instructions (for precautions see page 96). *Adults:* 1 fresh clove a day; not suitable for children under 6 years old.

Children (2-16 years old): adjust the adult dose downwards, depending on the age of the child – see Chapter 6.

Colds, prevention of

Make sure you eat a lot of fruit and vegetables and also plenty of garlic. There is no need to supplement your diet with vitamin C continually, but it is worth doing so if you feel that you have caught a cold. We are all more vulnerable to catching infections if our bodies are too hot or too cold (that's why Christmas shopping is an ideal terrain for a cold virus to spread, as shoppers pop in and out of shops getting excessively hot inside and cold outside), so dressing sensibly may ward off a lot of colds.

Avoiding crowded, air-conditioned areas is another simple way of minimising your chances of catching a cold, as is maintaining a distance from people who are already ill. Within a family, colds often spread through the use of the same cutlery or cups – just make sure you put them on a hot wash cycle or wash them extra well by hand.

Treatment options

- Drink one cup of elderflower tea every day throughout the winter season. *Adults:* 1 cup a day or 2-4 cups a day if you develop any symptoms.

- Take good-quality echinacea for 2 to 4 months (for precautions see page 98). *Adults:* 1-2ml diluted with some water, 3 times a day, tincture strength 1:5.

- Include raw garlic in your diet or take garlic capsules, according to the manufacturer's instructions (for precautions see page 96). *Adults:* 1 fresh clove a day; not suitable for children under 6 years old.

Children (2-16 years old): adjust the adult dose downwards, depending on the age of the child – see Chapter 6.

Colds, treatment of

If, in spite of all the preventative measures, you still develop a cold, you can minimise the symptoms with the help of herbs. Depending on the actual symptoms and their severity, you may need to use a combination of treatments. For more treatment options, look up specific symptoms, e.g. cough, sore throat or runny nose, separately in the next section of this chapter.

Treatment options

- Drink elderflower tea. *Adults:* 2-4 cups a day.

- Drink warming teas, e.g. lime tree flowers or ginger if you are shivering (for precautions see page 52). *Adults:* 1-3 cups a day.

- Reduce fever if it is above 38°C/100.4°F (see the Fever entry, page 108).

- Take fresh garlic with honey or garlic juice until symptoms improve (for precautions see page 96). *Adults:* 2-3 cloves a day or 1-3 teaspoons a day; not suitable for children under 6 years old.

- Take the anti-cold mix – see box overleaf.

- Take the mix for throat and chest infections – see box overleaf – if your cold is really bad, and you have either a sore throat or a cough, or both.

Children (2-16 years old): adjust the adult dose downwards, depending on the age of the child – see Chapter 6.

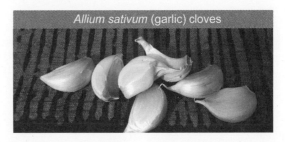
Allium sativum (garlic) cloves

ANTI-COLD MIX

Ingredients
- 50ml elderflower (tincture strength 1:5)
- 50ml stabilised garlic juice (for precautions see page 96)

To make
- Mix ingredients together.
- Pour into a clean, dark glass bottle.
- Label with the contents and the date.
- Store at room temperature for up to a year.

Adult dose: 5-10ml diluted with water, 1-3 times a day.

MIX FOR THROAT AND CHEST INFECTIONS

Ingredients
- 20ml mountain grape (tincture strength 1:2) (for precautions see page 102)
- 20ml thyme (tincture strength 1:2)
- 20ml elecampane (tincture strength 1:2)
- 40ml marshmallow root (tincture strength 1:5)

To make
- Mix ingredients together.
- Pour into a clean, dark glass bottle.
- Label with the contents and the date.
- Store at room temperature for up to a year.

Adult dose: 5ml diluted with some water, 2-3 times a day.

COUGH, DRY

A dry cough often results from a sore throat, but can also indicate a chest infection. The options listed below will reduce the frequency of coughing, especially at night. If the coughing wakes you up, take a teaspoon or two of marshmallow syrup, as it 'lubricates' the dry throat almost immediately.

Treatment options

- Take marshmallow syrup if your cough is caused by a dry, or a sore, throat. *Adults:* 8 teaspoonsful a day.

- Take thyme and liquorice syrup if you think that the infection has spread to your chest (for precautions see page 101). *Adults:* 1 teaspoonful 2-5 times a day.

- Use onion syrup (see page 98) to diminish the frequency of coughing, especially if you cough a lot at night. *Adults:* 4-5 teaspoonsful a day.

- Take echinacea tincture if your cough has been lingering for more than 10 days, but do not take it at the onset of the cough (for precautions see page 98). *Adults:* 1-2ml diluted with some water, 3 times a day, tincture strength 1:5.

- Take the tincture mix for a persistent cough – see box opposite.

Children (2-16 years old): adjust the adult dose downwards, depending on the age of the child – see Chapter 6.

MIX FOR A PERSISTENT COUGH

Ingredients
- 20ml thyme (tincture strength 1:2)
- 20ml liquorice (tincture strength 1:1) (for precautions see page 101)
- 20ml elecampane (tincture strength 1:2)
- 40ml ground ivy (tincture strength 1:2)

To make
- Mix ingredients together.
- Pour into a clean, dark glass bottle.
- Label with the contents and the date.
- Store at room temperature for up to a year.

Adult dose: 5ml diluted with some water, 2-3 times a day.

COUGH, PRODUCTIVE

Practitioner treatment is recommended for this condition.

A productive cough generally indicates the right response from your body: the airways are producing mucus as a reaction to the infection and coughing is a mechanism to remove the excess mucus. It is best not to suppress this mechanism but to aid it with the syrups that de-clog and disinfect the lungs. Yellow or green phlegm is a sign of a bacterial infection, and you may need professional help from a herbalist or antibiotics from your doctor.

Treatment options
- Take onion syrup (see page 98). *Adults:* 4-5 teaspoonsful a day.
- Take thyme and liquorice syrup (for precautions see page 101). *Adults:* 1 teaspoonful 2-5 times a day.
- Drink elderflower tea. *Adults:* 1-2 cups a day.
- Take the tincture mix for a persistent cough (see left) if your cough does not clear within 10 days.

Children (2-16 years old): adjust the adult dose downwards, depending on the age of the child – see Chapter 6.

EARACHE

Practitioner treatment is recommended for this condition.

This problem is most common in children. It is usually a sign of middle-ear infection, but can be a result of a growing wisdom tooth or a foreign body in the ear canal. The options below apply to mild infection and will be most effective right at the onset of the symptoms. Earache that does not improve within a day of treatment, gets progressively worse in spite of the treatment or is exceptionally severe needs professional attention.

Treatment options
- Apply St John's wort infused oil: soak one end of a piece of cotton wool in the oil, shake the excess so that it doesn't drip and insert it gently at the entrance of the ear canal (make sure you don't push it too far,

in order that you can easily extract it later). Leave in place for a few hours, ideally overnight. Use a smaller piece of cotton wool for children, and check periodically whether it is still in place.

- Apply calendula ointment **behind** the ear 2-3 times a day (for precautions see page 114).

- Take valerian tincture to reduce the pain. *Adults:* 5ml diluted with some water, 2-3 times a day, tincture strength 1:1. *Children (2-16 years old):* adjust the adult dose downwards, depending on the age of the child – see Chapter 6.

EAR INFECTIONS, RECURRENT

Practitioner treatment is recommended for this condition.

This problem affects mostly children and young adults.

Children with recurrent ear problems often respond dramatically to the removal of cow's milk from their diet (use goat's milk instead or talk to a nutritionist about other milk substitutes). Ice cream is a common culprit for causing ear problems, as is getting water in the ear at a swimming pool. Wearing a warm hat in cold weather is the best preventative measure, since having a cold head makes you vulnerable to infection.

Treatment options

- Take echinacea tincture for 1-3 months to improve the immune response (for precautions see page 98). *Adults:* 1-2ml diluted with some water, 2 times a day, tincture strength 1:5.

- Drink elderflower tea to reduce the formation of catarrh in the Eustachian tubes (passages that connect the inner ear to the throat). *Adults:* 1 cup a day.

Children (2-16 years old): adjust the adult dose downwards, depending on the age of the child – see Chapter 6.

- Apply calendula ointment **behind** the ear once a day (for precautions see page 114).

- Use St John's wort infused oil at the very onset of the symptoms (see Earache entry, page 107).

FEVER, REDUCING

Although fever is a natural defence mechanism of the body in fighting an infection, it can be very exhausting and can even cause fits in the young and loss of consciousness if allowed to run very high. In my view it makes sense to reduce fever, provided that you do not immediately resume your normal activity. A lowered temperature, as a result of either herbs or pharmaceuticals, does not mean that the infection has gone away – your body will be still busy fighting it for a few days and you should give it a chance to do the job properly. That means staying in bed, or at least at home for a day or two, until the temperature doesn't rise any more when you stop taking fever-reducing measures.

If the temperature creeps up above 38°C/100.4°F you may sometimes need to resort to aspirin or Paracetamol (but be aware that the use of Calpol in children has been recently linked with the increased incidence of childhood asthma and hay fever.[5]) The combination of elderflower tea and the conventional medicines above is more effective than either on its own when it comes to reducing a fever, so by using both you will need less of the pharmaceuticals.

Children can run a very high temperature very quickly, so you should monitor it with a thermometer every 2-3 hours and seek medical help if it goes above 39°C/102.2°F. Tepid sponging can be helpful: strip the child to his or her underwear and, using a sponge or a flannel, gently moisten the limbs and trunk with lukewarm water. Do not be tempted to use cold water – lukewarm water evaporates quicker and cools the body more effectively.

Treatment options

- Drink elderflower tea. *Adults:* 2-4 cups a day.

- Drink lime tree flower tea. *Adults:* 1-3 cups a day.

- Drink a tea for reducing fever – see box below.

TEA FOR REDUCING FEVER
Ingredients
- 50g dry elderflower
- 25g dry lime tree flower

To make
- Mix herbs thoroughly.
- Infuse 2 teaspoons of the mix in a cupful of freshly boiled water for 10 minutes. Strain and drink warm. You can add honey to this tea.

Adult dose: 1-3 cups a day.

Children (2-16 years old): adjust the adult dose downwards, depending on the age of the child – see Chapter 6.

FLU

Practitioner treatment is recommended for this condition.

The difference between an ordinary cold and flu is a question of severity of symptoms. Flu is caused by specific influenza viruses, strains of which can be quite virulent. People with flu usually experience high fever, severe coughing, muscle ache, headache and nausea. They often feel very weak, virtually unable to drag themselves out of bed. Flu usually lasts longer than a cold, and can leave you exhausted and depressed for weeks afterwards. Flu can be a serious disease and requires vigorous treatment.

The use of echinacea once the flu has already started is controversial, according to current research,[6] and I would not recommend doing so.

Treatment options

- If coughing is a prominent feature, use remedies that are antiseptic for the lungs (see Bronchitis and Cough entries, pages 103-4 and 106-7) .

- Keep an eye on the temperature and, if necessary, bring it down by measures described in the Fever entry, page 108.

- Take the antiviral mix, which combines 3 herbs with antiviral properties – see box overleaf.

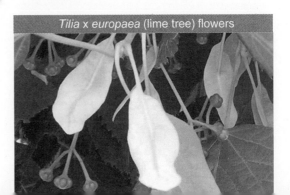
Tilia x europaea (lime tree) flowers

ANTIVIRAL MIX

Ingredients

- 50ml elderflower (tincture strength 1:5)
- 30ml garlic juice (for precautions see page 96)
- 20ml propolis (tincture strength 1:10) (for precautions see page 99)

To make

- Mix ingredients together.
- Pour into a clean, dark glass bottle.
- Label with the contents and the date.
- Store at room temperature for up to a year.

Adult dose: 5ml diluted with some water, 2-3 times a day.

Children: adjust the adult dose downwards, depending on the age of the child – see Chapter 6.

Note: Not suitable for children under 6 years old because of garlic and propolis.

HAY FEVER

Practitioner treatment is recommended for this condition.

This is a condition that is tricky to treat successfully at home, but many people seem to be able to lessen their sensitivity to pollen by eating local honey every day and well in advance of the pollen season.

Treatment options

- Drink elderflower tea, starting a month before the pollen season and continuing throughout. *Adults:* 1-2 cups a day.

- Drink eyebright tea before and during the pollen season. *Adults:* 1-2 cups a day.

Children (2-16 years old): adjust the adult dose downwards, depending on the age of the child – see Chapter 6.

SINUSITIS

Practitioner treatment is recommended for this condition.

Sinusitis usually follows a bad cold with a runny nose and a lot of catarrh. The symptoms are: blocked nose, green or yellow discharge from the nose, dull pain above the eyebrows or below the eye sockets, and slight fever.

Sinusitis can be quite tricky to treat yourself, especially if it is chronic (long-lasting). If you do not respond to the measures below, see a medical herbalist.

Treatment options

- Eat lots of fresh garlic or take garlic juice (for precautions see page 96). *Adults:* 2-3 cloves a day; or 1 teaspoonful of garlic juice 2 times a day. Not suitable for children under 6 years old.

- Inhale steam from tea tree essential oil and hot water under a towel. *Adults:* 5 drops in a large bowl of hot water.

- Massage tea tree essential oil into the painful areas over the eyebrows and on the cheeks (for precautions see page 118). *Adults:* dilute 5 drops of the essential oil in 10ml of almond oil, massage 1-3 times a day.

Children (3-16 years old): adjust the adult dose

downwards, depending on the age of the child – see Chapter 6.

SORE THROAT

If your throat is just red and swollen you are probably suffering from a viral infection, in which case use the normal measures applicable to any cold, but you should use a gargle (see below) as well. If your tonsils have white spots on them it is a bacterial infection, which may have to be treated with antibiotics. However, a natural antibiotic in the form of propolis spray or lozenges can combat many such infections.

Some texts recommend eating ice cream to reduce throat pain; I cannot see the logic in this advice – the relief from pain is short-lived and the soreness comes back with a vengeance!

Treatment options

- Drink elderflower tea. *Adults:* 2-4 cups a day.

- Gargle with warm sage tea. *Adults:* half a cup 2-4 times a day.

- Gargle with one of the gargles on page 63.

- Apply propolis spray to the throat or take propolis lozenges (for precautions see page 99). *Adults:* spray 3-4 times a day or 1-4 lozenges a day.

- Take fresh garlic with honey or drink garlic juice (for precautions see page 96). *Adults:* 1-2 cloves a day; or 1 teaspoonful of garlic juice 1-2 times a day.

Children (2-16 years old): adjust the adult dose downwards, depending on the age of the child – see Chapter 6.

TONSILLITIS

Practitioner treatment is recommended for this condition.

Tonsillitis can be distinguished from an ordinary sore throat both by white spots on the tonsils, which become very tender and swollen, and by a high temperature. See Sore throat entry, left.

Treatment options

- Use propolis spray or take propolis lozenges. Children are unlikely to accept a propolis spray, but propolis lozenges are quite tasty; use the manufacturer's instructions to adjust the dose for children. For precautions see page 99. *Adults:* spray 3-4 times a day; or 2-4 lozenges a day.

- Prepare and take an antibacterial mix for tonsillitis – see box overleaf.

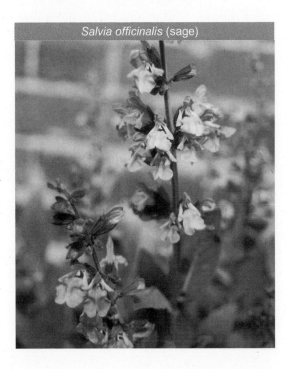
Salvia officinalis (sage)

ANTIBACTERIAL MIX FOR TONSILLITIS

Ingredients
- 20ml thyme (tincture strength 1:2)
- 20ml propolis (tincture strength 1:10) (for precautions see page 99)
- 30ml garlic juice (for precautions see page 96)
- 30ml mountain grape (tincture strength 1:2) (for precautions see page 102)

To make
- Mix ingredients together.
- Pour into a clean, dark glass bottle.
- Label with the contents and the date.
- Store at room temperature for up to a year.

Adult dose: 5ml diluted with some water, 3 times a day until the symptoms improve, then 2.5ml, 3 times a day for 2 days.

Children: adjust the adult dose downwards, depending on the age of the child – see Chapter 6.

Note: Not suitable for children under 6 years old.

WHEN AND WHY YOU SHOULD SEE A PROFESSIONAL MEDICAL HERBALIST

- Asthma: herbal treatment can greatly reduce the need for inhalers. The treatment will be highly individualised, depending on the type and severity of your asthma.

- Bronchitis, chronic: this mostly affects older people, and needs an individual approach and the right combination of antibacterial and anti-inflammatory herbs.

- Chronic fatigue syndrome: also called ME, this is a profound tiredness often following a viral infection or glandular fever. It can be very successfully treated with individually prescribed herbs; the treatment will depend on your case history and constitution.

- Hay fever: like eczema and asthma, this requires an individual approach combined with adjustments to the diet and the patient's environment.

- Sinusitis, chronic: this usually requires a long-term treatment lasting a few months and will depend on your health history.

THE FOLLOWING SYMPTOMS WARRANT SEEING A HEALTH PROFESSIONAL WITHOUT DELAY

- Pain in the chest when coughing.

- High temperature (above 39°C/102°F) and dry/productive cough.

- Difficulty in breathing.

- Painful enlargement of the glands around the neck.

- Flu-like symptoms combined with a stiff neck and constant, severe headache.

- Persistent cough lasting for weeks.

- Persistent cough accompanied by night sweats.

Chapter 15
The skin

Skin is our interface with the outside world. It is the largest organ in our body and it is intimately connected with our vascular and nervous systems. While superficial skin problems can be dealt most effectively by external treatment, many chronic skin problems relate to deeper layers of the skin and hence respond better to internal treatment.

INTERNAL TREATMENT

Herbalists always make links between the appearance of the skin and what is happening inside the body, and for them treating skin problems with internal medicine is the most logical step. Skin diseases often result from very complex interactions between our immune system, our hormonal system, our diet and the state of our nerves – so it follows that a complex approach and a complex prescription are needed for complicated problems such as eczema, psoriasis, acne or acne rosacea. Careful observation is often needed to see what triggers certain problems.

EXTERNAL APPLICATIONS

On the other hand, most of the common, everyday skin problems such as cuts, burns, stings, etc. can be effectively treated with specific herbal preparations for external use that greatly enhance the rate at which skin heals.

DOSAGE FOR EXTERNAL REMEDIES

There is no distinction between adult or child external treatment when the area of affected skin is small. If a large area of body is affected in children, please consult a medical herbalist before applying large amounts of cream containing essential oils. Essential oils are absorbed partially into the bloodstream from the cream, and therefore caution is needed with small children.

CAUTION WITH EYE TREATMENT

Some of the ailments of eyes, scalp and hair can be easily tackled at home, but extra caution should be exercised in the case of eyes. If you are not entirely confident that you are applying the right treatment to your eyes it is best to consult your GP.

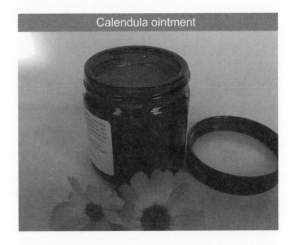
Calendula ointment

MUST-HAVE HERBS

The herbs in this section are listed in order of usefulness.

CALENDULA

> **Caution needed** if allergic to plants of the *Compositae* family.

Uses

Otherwise known as marigold, calendula is *the* treatment for the skin. It is antibacterial, antiviral and anti-fungal. It promotes skin cell division and hence the healing of any skin injury. It is also anti-inflammatory. Calendula can be used in any situation where the skin has been broken, either through injury or disease. Its main uses include the treatment of cuts, grazes, sunburn, heat burns, insect stings, various skin rashes and nappy rash. Unless you are allergic to calendula, you can try it on virtually any skin problem except for bruising, where comfrey would be better.

Unfortunately, some people who suffer from multiple allergies may also be allergic to calendula. In my experience, this precludes them from using calendula internally, and some cases of eczema can become worse after the application of calendula ointment on the affected areas. However, the same people can still use calendula for cuts or burns without adverse effects.

How to use

You can use calendula as an ointment, cream, infused oil, poultice or compress, depending on the problem. It is easy to make your own calendula ointment and I recommend that you do so (see Chapter 26) – home-made ointment will be far superior to anything that you can buy over the counter.

Dosage

This is specific to the problem: see individual entries in the next section of this chapter.

COMFREY

> **Warning:** Use only for external treatment.

Uses

Comfrey is very similar in its action to calendula, as it promotes skin cell division and the healing of skin injuries. It is generally less allergenic and is therefore suitable for people who cannot tolerate calendula or chamomile. It is best in cases of 'mixed' injuries, where there is some bruising combined with an open wound. Internal treatment with comfrey is not recommended at present.

How to use

You can apply this herb in the form of cream, ointment, infused oil, poultice or compress.

Dosage

This is specific to the problem: see individual entries in the next section of this chapter.

CHAMOMILE

> **Caution needed** if allergic to plants of the *Compositae* family.

Uses

This herb can be used as an internal or external remedy for many skin complaints. A very small proportion of people can be severely allergic to chamomile, especially when applied to the skin. If you have never used it before, try it first on a small patch of skin for a few days before applying it to a larger area. Chamomile has an anti-inflammatory action for skin problems and can therefore be used for any conditions where inflammation is a feature: acne, swellings of various origins, dry eczema, insect bites, sore eyes, etc.

How to use
You can apply it as a cream, poultice or compress.

Dosage
External applications: this is specific to the problem; see individual entries in the next section of this chapter.
Internal dose for adults: 3-10ml a day, 1-3 times a day, tincture strength 1:5.
Internal dose for children (2-16 years old): adjust the adult dose downwards, depending on the age of the child – see Chapter 6.

THYME

Warning: Do not use essential oils for external applications in pregnancy or for children under 3 years old without consulting a specialist.

All other thyme preparations are safe for small children and in pregnancy.

Uses
Thyme can be used externally to treat skin infections, sunburn or a variety of itchy conditions; for instance, it is an excellent remedy for treating itchy conditions of the genital area. It is the remedy to try on fungal infections, either by itself or mixed with other anti-fungal herbs. It also makes a good skin disinfectant for small injuries.

How to use
You can use thyme externally either as tincture, infusion, compress or thyme essential oil. Tinctures or infusions applied directly to the skin with cotton wool are called lotions. Tincture should be diluted slightly to avoid stinging: 10ml of tincture with at least 50ml of water.

Dosage
External applications: this is specific to the problem – see individual entries in the next section of this chapter.

OPTIONAL HERBS

ECHINACEA (PURPLE CONEFLOWER)

Caution needed if allergic to plants of the *Compositae* family.

Uses
Although mostly known as a general immune stimulant, echinacea can be useful in some cases of skin disease as an external application. Native Americans traditionally used it for the treatment of various wounds.

How to use
You can use diluted echinacea tincture for disinfecting cuts and grazes, or you can take it internally if you suffer from a chronic skin problem such as acne or eczema – but make sure you start on a minimal dose to avoid any possible worsening of the condition.

Dosage

Adults: 1-2ml diluted with some water, 1-3 times a day, tincture strength 1:5.

Children (2-16 years old): adjust the internal adult dose downwards, depending on the age of the child – see Chapter 6.

EYEBRIGHT

Uses

The name of this herb reflects its use – eyebright is *the* herb for external eye problems. It can be used for eye irritation, tiredness, eye watering, mild conjunctivitis, puffiness and itching.

How to use

Eye irritation that is a feature of hay fever responds best to internal treatment with eyebright tincture; other conditions can be treated with an eye bath containing a tiny amount of the tincture (see Conjunctivitis entry later in this chapter).

Dosage

External applications: this is specific to the problem; see individual entries in the next section of this chapter.

Internal dose for adults: 1-2ml diluted with some water, 2-3 times a day, tincture strength 1:2.

Internal dose for children (2-16 years old): adjust the adult dose downwards, depending on the age of the child – see Chapter 6.

LAVENDER

Warning: Do not use essential oils for external applications in pregnancy or for children under 3 years old without consulting a specialist.

Uses

Lavender is another herbal antiseptic, not as strong as tea tree (see page 118) but less irritating to the skin. It is also mildly anti-inflammatory. Lavender essential oil is the only essential oil that I would add to eczema cream; in my experience the others sooner or later cause skin irritation.

How to use

Lavender essential oil should be used for external applications mixed into a cream – see box below.

ANTISEPTIC AND HEALING CREAM (NO.1)

Ingredients

- 10-20 drops lavender essential oil (for precautions see above)
- 50g calendula or comfrey cream (for precautions see page 114)

To make

- Mix well and transfer to a clean, dark glass jar, making sure that there are no air pockets left. Store for up to 12 months.

Adults and children over 3 years old: apply to the affected skin 1-3 times a day.

Note: this cream may sting temporarily if the skin is broken.

Mountain grape

Warning: Do not use when pregnant or breastfeeding.

Uses
This herb provides a basis for the treatment of chronic (long-lasting) skin diseases such as psoriasis, acne, acne rosacea, eczema and boils. Mountain grape has anti-inflammatory and antimicrobial actions that make it very useful for skin problems.

How to take
I recommend using it for internal treatment in the form of tincture.

Dosage
Adults: 1-2.5ml diluted with some water, 1-3 times a day, tincture strength 1:2.
Children (2-16 years old): adjust the internal adult dose downwards, depending on the age of the child – see Chapter 6.

Nettle leaf

Uses
Nettle leaf is an example of a herb that improves the detoxification of the body. As such it is useful in skin conditions that are allergic in nature, such as eczema or urticaria (hives).

How to take
Nettle leaf can be taken as a tea or as a tincture.

Dosage
Adults: 1-2 cups of tea a day; or 0.7-2ml diluted with some water, 1-3 times a day, tincture strength 1:2.

Children (2-16 years old): adjust the internal adult dose downwards, depending on the age of the child – see Chapter 6.

Red clover

Uses
Red clover can be used internally for most skin disorders. It is gently detoxifying and does not exacerbate any existing problems (some stronger herbal detoxifiers can cause temporary worsening). You can include it in any internal mix of tea or tincture for acne, eczema or psoriasis.

Combinations
Red clover mixes well with yellow dock and/or mountain grape.

How to take
As tincture or as tea.

Dosage
Adults: 1-2ml diluted with some water, 1-3 times a day, tincture strength 1:2; or 1-2 cups of tea a day.
Children (2-16 years old): adjust the internal adult dose downwards, depending on the age of the child – see Chapter 6.

Ribwort plantain

Uses
This herb is a general soother for inflamed skin conditions, for instance eczema. It also enhances the natural ability of the skin to heal. It is a very gentle herb that is suitable for people with multiple allergies.

How to use

Ribwort plantain can be taken on its own or combined with other skin remedies for internal treatment, either as a tea or as a tincture. It can also be applied externally to weeping and inflamed skin, as a compress or poultice. For this purpose use a strong tea or freshly squeezed juice.

Dosage

Adults: 1-3 cups of tea a day; or 1-2ml diluted with some water, 1-3 times a day, tincture strength 1:2.

Children (2-16 years old): adjust the internal adult dose downwards, depending on the age of the child – see Chapter 6.

TEA TREE

Warning: Do not use essential oils for external applications in pregnancy or for children under 3 years old without consulting a specialist.

Uses

Tea tree is one of the strongest herbal antiseptics for external use. I recommend using it for skin infections, fungal or bacterial.

How to use

As an essential oil, I do not recommend using tea tree neat on the skin because it can cause local skin irritation. My preferred use is in the form of a cream – see box, above right.

ANTISEPTIC AND HEALING CREAM (NO.2)

Ingredients
- 20 drops of tea tree essential oil (for precautions see below left)
- 50g of calendula or comfrey cream (for precautions see page 114)

To make
- Mix well and transfer to a clean, dark glass jar, making sure that there are no air pockets left. Store for up to 12 months.

Adults and children over 3 years old: apply to the affected skin 1-3 times a day.
Note: this cream may sting temporarily if the skin is broken.

VALERIAN

Uses

Valerian, being a strong relaxant, makes a very useful addition to the treatment of skin problems that are exacerbated by stress.

How to use

Take valerian tincture on a daily basis for 1-2 months; use the minimal dosage.

Dosage

Adults: 0.3-1ml diluted with some water, 1-3 times a day, tincture strength 1:1.

Children (2-16 years old): adjust the internal adult dose downwards, depending on the age of the child – see Chapter 6.

YELLOW DOCK

Warning: Use only small doses if breast-feeding.

Uses
Yellow dock is another general detoxifier, which is especially useful whenever skin problems are made worse by constipation (yellow dock is a gentle laxative). It can be used for eczema, acne and psoriasis.

Combinations
It combines well with red clover, mountain grape and ribwort plantain.

How to take
Yellow dock is a fairly strong-acting herb, so it should be introduced gradually, at the lower end of the recommended dose. If you mix it with other herbs, yellow dock should constitute no more than about 10-20% of the mix. It can be taken as a tea but has a rather strong taste, so it really needs to be mixed with other dry herbs, for instance, red clover and ribwort plantain (see page 117).

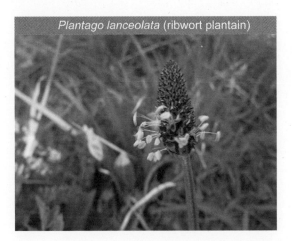
Plantago lanceolata (ribwort plantain)

Dosage
Adults: 1-2ml diluted with water, 1-3 times a day, tincture strength 1:5.
Children (2-16 years old): adjust the internal adult dose downwards, depending on the age of the child – see Chapter 6.

SPECIFIC AILMENTS AFFECTING THE SKIN & HERBS THAT CAN HELP

ACNE

Practitioner treatment is recommended for this condition.

Acne can be very troublesome for teenagers, and sometimes it persists into adulthood. It may require prolonged treatment, sometimes with herbs that can influence the hormones involved. The measures below can be tried singly or in combination, depending on how severe the acne is. If it is an occasional single spot, just treat it with external remedies. If it is quite a few spots, take internal treatment – again, either singly or combined, and also use external remedies. The internal treatment for acne often needs to be ongoing for months or even years to bring sustained results. Supplementing with zinc will aid skin healing, although it may be necessary to improve the whole diet – avoid chocolate, coffee and alcohol.

Treatment options
- Drink chamomile tea on a daily basis – it is the simplest measure but surprisingly effective; the key is to drink it every day! For precautions see page 114. *Adults:* 1-2

cups a day – use 2 teaspoonsful of loose herbs or 2 tea bags per cup.

- Take propolis capsules daily if you get a lot of painful spots that resemble small boils (for precautions see page 99). *Adults:* you need to take the equivalent of 2-3g of propolis a day, starting with 1g and increasing to 3g if your symptoms are severe.

- Drink the tea for improving skin problems – see box, right.

- Take the tincture mix for skin disorders – see box below.

Teenagers (11-16 years old): adjust the internal adult dose downwards, depending on the age of the teenager – see Chapter 6.

TEA FOR IMPROVING SKIN PROBLEMS

Ingredients
- 20g dry yellow dock (for precautions see page 119)
- 40g dry red clover flower
- 40g dry ribwort plantain

To make
- Mix herbs thoroughly.
- Infuse 2 teaspoonsful of the mix in a cupful of freshly boiled water for 10 minutes. Strain and drink warm. You can add honey to this tea.

Adult dose: 1 cup a day until the symptoms improve, then half a cup for 2-4 months.

MIX FOR SKIN DISORDERS

Ingredients
- 20ml yellow dock (tincture strength 1:5) (for precautions see page 119)
- 20ml red clover (tincture strength 1:2)
- 20ml mountain grape (tincture strength 1:2) (for precautions see page 117)
- 40ml ribwort plantain (tincture strength 1:2)

To make
- Mix ingredients together.
- Pour into a clean, dark glass bottle.
- Label with the contents and the date.
- Store at room temperature for up to a year.

Adult dose: 5ml diluted with some water 3 times a day until the symptoms improve, then 5ml a day to maintain the improvement for 2-4 months.

- Wipe the affected areas of the skin with witch hazel water after washing. *Adults and teenagers:* 1-2 times a day, but if you find it too drying do it every other day.

- Dab tea tree essential oil neat on the developing spots (For precautions see page 118.) *Adults and teenagers:* twice a day.

- Apply neat calendula tincture directly to the spots with a cotton bud: if you start doing it as soon as you feel a spot is beginning to develop, you should be able to prevent it from growing altogether. (For precautions see page 114.) *Adults and teenagers:* 2-5 times a day.

- Big spots respond well to repeated application of calendula ointment (gently rub on a small amount); try to apply it as soon as you develop a painful swelling, and keep reapplying it every couple of hours or so. (For precautions see page 114.) *Adults and teenagers:* 3-6 times a day.

ATHLETE'S FOOT

Athlete's foot is a fungal infection that usually 'sits' between the toes but can also infect toenails or spread to other parts of the body. Fungal infections thrive in an extra-warm, moist environment with little air – wearing closed-toe shoes all day, especially in summer, provides perfect conditions. Whenever you can, let your feet 'breathe' to prevent the occurrence in the first place, and wear woollen or cotton socks. The measures below will help to heal the painful splits that athlete's foot often leads to and will reduce the itching. Unfortunately, it is very easy to get reinfected with the fungus again as the spores can persist in shoes, socks and towels. Change your socks every day and do not share your towels with other members of the family. Try not to wear the same shoes every day, to prevent moisture build-up.

Treatment options

- Apply the anti-fungal ointment – see box on the right.

- Once the infection clears up, you can use the above ointment as a preventative measure. *Adults and children over 3 years old:* apply a small amount between the toes for a few months once a day.

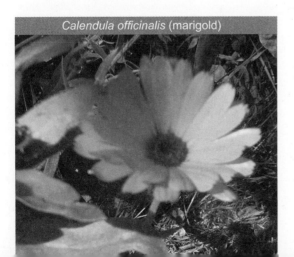
Calendula officinalis (marigold)

ANTI-FUNGAL OINTMENT

Ingredients
- 50g calendula ointment or cream (for precautions see page 114)
- 10 drops of tea tree essential oil (for precautions see page 118)
- 10 drops of thyme essential oil (for precautions see page 115)

To make
- Mix well.
- Transfer to a clean, dark glass jar making sure that there are no air pockets left. Store for up to 12 months.

Adults and children over 3 years old: apply to the infected areas morning and evening, after a bath or shower.

Note: This cream may sting temporarily if the skin is split.

BOILS

Practitioner treatment is recommended for this condition. If you are not confident that the treatment is working, see a doctor, as the bacteria from the boil can infect blood and lead to septicaemia, which is a potentially life-threatening condition.

This condition is quite rare nowadays, as people live much more hygienic lives than they used to and have better nutrition, both of which help to prevent skin infection. However, people with lowered immunity or nutritional deficiencies can still be prone to having boils, so it is worth knowing how to treat them at home. The idea is to bring the boil to a head and then get rid of the accumulated pus by gentle pressure; healing usually occurs rapidly once the pus is removed.

Treatment options

- Make a warm poultice from 1-2 tablespoons of ground linseed and proceed as with the paste for drawing boils (see right).

- Take propolis capsules or tincture (for precautions see page 99). *Adults:* 1-2 ml, 2-3 times a day, tincture strength 1:10; or capsules should be equivalent to 3g of propolis a day divided into 3 portions.

- Take echinacea tincture (for precautions see page 115). *Adults:* 1-2 ml 2-3 times a day, tincture strength 1:5.

- Apply the paste for drawing boils – see box, right.

Children (2-16 years old): adjust the internal adult dose downwards, depending on the age of the child – see Chapter 6.

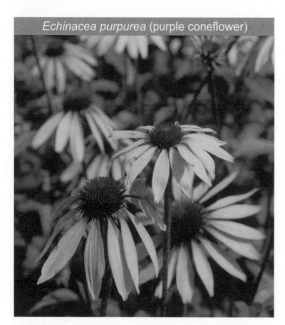
Echinacea purpurea (purple coneflower)

PASTE FOR DRAWING BOILS

Ingredients

- 1 heaped teaspoonful of marshmallow root powder
- a little boiled water
- 5 drops of tea tree essential oil (for precautions see page 118)
- 5 drops of lavender or thyme essential oil (for precautions see pages 81 and 115)
- 1-2g of calendula ointment (for precautions see page 114)

To make

- Mix all the ingredients to a paste consistency.

To apply

- Put the paste on to a gauze dressing, press gently against the boil and fix in place with a large plaster or bandage. Change this dressing every few hours until there is a definite white head at the centre of the boil. Gently pressing around the boil should result in bursting it; you need to keep on gently squeezing until all the pus is gone.
- Afterwards, dress with some calendula ointment and a plaster.
- Repeat the whole procedure if the boil starts swelling up again.

BURNS

Ordinary burns usually happen at home while cooking, using electrical appliances (mostly ironing) or using fireplaces. If your burn is extensive, seek medical advice. Otherwise, place the injured area under running cold water as soon as possible and keep it there until the pain subsides (sometimes it is easier to plunge a burnt limb in a sink filled with cold water). Only then use the measures below.

Treatment options

- Apply a thin layer of calendula ointment (for precautions see page 114). Do not cover the burn if the skin is unbroken.

- If the skin is broken you may need to cover the area once the pain subsides. Put a good layer of calendula cream on a plaster or gauze before covering the burn. This will stop the cover sticking to the wound and will speed up the healing. For precautions see page 114.

- If you have no calendula cream, soak the burned area in a cold calendula infusion for 5-10 minutes or apply a cold calendula infusion compress. For precautions see page 114.

COLD SORE

A cold sore is a viral infection which often goes with a cold or flu. It is said that once you have it, it will keep recurring, because the virus that is causing it persists in the nerve cells. However, repeated treatment with calendula seems to diminish the frequency of eruptions. The ointment must be of the highest quality (see Chapter 26 for making your own).

Treatment options

- Apply calendula ointment as soon as you feel the cold sore coming, and keep applying small amounts every hour or so; this should stop the cold sore from developing. For precautions see page 114.

- If the cold sore has already erupted, keep

applying calendula ointment 3-5 times a day. For precautions see page 114.

- Take elderflower tea for its antiviral properties. *Adults:* 2-3 cups a day.

Children (2-16 years old): adjust the internal adult dose downwards, depending on the age of the child – see Chapter 6.

- Apply lemon balm cream for cold sores – see box below.

LEMON BALM CREAM FOR COLD SORES

Ingredients

- 50g calendula or comfrey cream (for precautions see page 114)
- 20 drops of lemon balm essential oil (for precautions see page 53)

To make

- Mix well.
- Transfer to a clean, dark glass jar, making sure that there are no air pockets left
- Store for up to 12 months.

Adults and children over 3 years old: apply thinly to the cold sore every 2-3 hours during daytime until the sore is gone.

Note: this cream may sting temporarily.

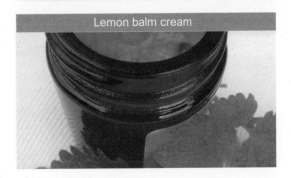
Lemon balm cream

Conjunctivitis

Practitioner treatment is recommended for this condition.

Conjunctivitis is best treated by a doctor, but a mild eye irritation can be treated at home. The most successful treatment is provided by an eye bath made with saline solution and a herbal tincture. You can get sterile saline from the optician or chemist, usually in the form of contact-lens solution (make sure it is just saline; the solutions with enzymes or other additives should not be used). I do not recommend using water for eye baths as it does sting. If both eyes are affected, use a fresh eye bath for each eye. Always sterilise an eye bath before and after use with boiling water, as eye infections can be very contagious. If the symptoms persist or become worse after trying the measures below, seek medical help.

Treatment options

- Make an eye bath: use 30ml of sterile saline plus **one drop** of eyebright tincture. *Adults and children over 5 years old:* bathe the affected eye 1-3 times a day for 10-20 seconds each time.

- Make an eye bath: use 30ml of sterile saline plus **½ teaspoon** of filtered eyebright tea; the tea should be brewed in the normal way and strained through a dense cloth or coffee filter. *Adults and children over 5 years old:* bathe the affected eye 1-3 times a day for 10-20 seconds each time.

- If the eyelids are sore and swollen, apply an eyebright compress – see box, right.

EYEBRIGHT COMPRESS

Ingredients
- 2 teaspoonsful of eyebright tincture
- 50ml of warm freshly boiled water

or

- ½ cup of freshly infused eyebright tea

To apply (it is best to lie down for this treatment)
- Mix the tincture with the water or strain the tea.
- Soak 2 pieces of cotton wool in the liquid, and squeeze out the excess.
- Apply the pieces to the eyelids.

Adult dose: apply the compress for 5-10 minutes, then re-soak the cotton wool pieces and apply again (the liquid should feel warm to the eyelids).
Children and babies: use **cool** eyebright tea, **not the tincture**, and apply for only 1-3 minutes.

Cradle cap

Cradle cap is regarded as a form of dermatitis, but it is unclear what the cause is. Although unsightly, cradle cap will eventually clear by itself. Sometimes it can still be present in older children, even in teenagers. Cradle cap is not itchy and doesn't bother babies, so I think it is generally best left alone unless it is exceptionally thick and widespread. When trying the treatment below, make sure that the olive oil doesn't get into the baby's eyes; you need only a small amount of oil. Olive oil should be used in preference to other oils as it hardly ever causes an allergic reaction.

Treatment options

- Apply olive oil to the scalp in the evening, leave it there for the night and then gently wash it off the next day – the dry skin scales should come off quite easily during washing or with gentle brushing afterwards; don't pull off stubborn scales that seem to be stuck, but repeat the treatment a few days later.

CUTS, GRAZES AND WOUNDS

Always make sure that you clean any debris or dirt from the wound as far as possible before you apply any treatment. Run water from the tap over the cut if you can, or gently wipe the wound with cotton wool soaked in clean water. Disinfect in the manner described below. If the cut is small leave it exposed to the air, but if it is large or vulnerable to getting dirty or being knocked, cover it with a plaster. Obviously, check the wound if any discomfort develops.

Treatment options

All these options are suitable for children over 2 years old.

- After cleaning, you can disinfect with any neat or slightly diluted herbal tincture (it will be alcohol that will do the most disinfecting and it will sting!); many herbs are antibacterial and you can choose from the following for stronger disinfecting action: thyme, calendula (for precautions see page 114), mountain grape, barberry, echinacea (for precautions see page 117, 51 and 115), or propolis (for precautions see page 99).

- If the cut is bleeding heavily, apply diluted yarrow tincture or yarrow juice (see page 40). For precautions see page 34.

- Apply a small amount of calendula ointment around the cut if you intend to leave it open to the air (for precautions see page 114).

- If you intend to cover the injury, apply calendula ointment liberally and leave the dressing in place for 24 hours. Repeat until the cut is healed. For precautions see page 114.

- If the wound is difficult to clean and you are worried that it may become infected, you can use Antiseptic and healing cream No.2 (see page 118).

DANDRUFF / ITCHY SCALP

Dandruff and itchy scalp often go together. The causes of dandruff are not clear, but some contributing factors include sensitivity to shampoos or other hair products, seborrhoeic eczema and mild fungal infection. If you have any spots or sores on the scalp you must consult a doctor for a proper diagnosis.

For the treatment of common dandruff and/or itchiness I suggest making your own shampoo from a shampoo base that is free from sodium lauryl sulphate, and a combination of tinctures. Rinsing or rubbing the scalp with specific herbal teas can also help.

Treatment options

All these options are suitable for children over 2 years old.

- After washing your hair, add calendula tea to the final rinse (you will need to infuse a substantial amount, about 1 litre). For precautions see page 114.

- Rub calendula or thyme tea directly on to the itchy scalp on a daily basis for a month or until the symptoms improve (use a small piece of cotton wool to apply the tea to the scalp). For precautions see page 114.

- Use your own home-mixed herbal shampoo for a few months – see boxes.

HOME-MIXED HERBAL SHAMPOO (NO.1)

Ingredients
- 120ml mild shampoo base (available from many herbal retailers)
- 20ml chamomile tincture (for precautions see page 114)
- 20ml rosemary tincture
- 20ml thyme tincture
- 20ml hops tincture

To make
- Mix the ingredients together in a measuring jug.
- Decant into a glass or plastic bottle. The shampoo will be quite runny.

Adults and children: use as an ordinary shampoo but lather your hair only once, then rinse thoroughly; you can use this shampoo on a daily basis.

Note: your herbal shampoo can theoretically be made with strong infusions instead of tinctures, but unless you use the shampoo quickly it may go off.

HOME-MIXED HERBAL SHAMPOO (NO.2)

Ingredients
- 120ml mild shampoo base (available from many herbal retailers)
- 20ml calendula tincture (for precautions see page 114)
- 20ml horsetail tincture
- 20ml horse chestnut tincture
- 20ml lemon balm tincture
- 1-2 drops of tea tree essential oil (for precautions see page 118)

To make
- Mix the ingredients together in a measuring jug.
- Decant into a glass or plastic bottle. The shampoo will be quite runny.

Adults and children: use as an ordinary shampoo but lather your hair only once, then rinse thoroughly; you can use this shampoo on a daily basis.

Note: your herbal shampoo can theoretically be made with strong infusions instead of tinctures, but unless you use the shampoo quickly it may go off.

ECZEMA

Practitioner treatment is recommended for this condition.

Eczema is very difficult to treat, as it is a condition caused by many contributing factors. Before trying a specific treatment you must look at any provoking factors and try to eliminate them as much as possible.

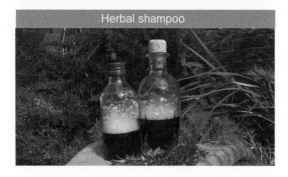
Herbal shampoo

Triggers for eczema include:

- dietary items – the most common are cow's milk and dairy products, chocolate, oranges, fizzy drinks, wheat and food additives; less common are bananas, tomatoes and spicy food.

- environmental items – biological washing powders, household chemicals, cosmetics, synthetic fabrics and dust mites.

- stress.

Careful observation is needed to link particular events with eczema flare-ups. Often a selective exclusion of the most allergenic items is enough to clear eczema completely. If that doesn't work you can try both internal and external treatment, but you must proceed very carefully as many herbs have the potential for making eczema worse. Internal treatment usually consists of anti-inflammatory and detoxifying herbs; sometimes an immune modulator and a relaxant for the nervous system are also called for. External treatment consists of a healing cream, but you must be very cautious and try each cream on a small area to begin with. It is not uncommon to develop a reaction to a cream that was working very well to begin with, and sometimes you may need two or three different creams used in rotation.

Treatment options

- Apply calendula ointment/cream to the affected areas (for precautions see page 114). *Adults and children over 2 years old:* 1-2 times a day.

- Apply either of the antiseptic and healing creams (see pages 116 and 118), especially if the eczema gets infected.

- A soothing treatment, especially for babies and small children, is an 'oat bath'. It is a little bit messy but calming to the skin. You need an old stocking or pair of tights, or a piece of muslin cloth, which you can fill with a couple of tablespoons of ordinary porridge oats. Tie it tightly so that the oat grains don't escape, then swish it in the bath water until the water acquires a milky look (or soak it for a few minutes until the oats release their milky contents). Adding a few drops of hemp seed oil to the bath will make it even more soothing. Do this every other day.

- Try one of the mixes for eczema (internal use) – see boxes below and overleaf.

MIX FOR ECZEMA (NO.1)

Ingredients

- 20ml liquorice (tincture strength 1:1) (for precautions see page 101)
- 30ml calendula (tincture strength 1:2) (for precautions see page 114)
- 50ml ribwort plantain (tincture strength 1:2)

To make

- Mix ingredients together.
- Pour into a clean, dark glass bottle.
- Label with the contents and the date.
- Store at room temperature for up to a year.

Adult dose: 5ml, diluted with some water, 2-3 times a day.

Children (2-16 years old): adjust the internal adult dose downwards, depending on the age of the child – see Chapter 6.

MIX FOR ECZEMA (NO.2)

Ingredients
- 30ml chamomile (tincture strength 1:2) (for precautions see page 114)
- 30ml dandelion root (tincture strength 1:2) (for precautions see page 51)
- 40ml ribwort plantain (tincture strength 1:2)

To make
- Mix ingredients together.
- Pour into a clean, dark glass bottle.
- Label with the contents and the date.
- Store at room temperature for up to a year.

Adult dose: 5ml, diluted with some water 2-3 times a day.

ITCHY SKIN

Skin can itch due to many problems – some visible, such as eczema; some less obvious, such as stress or liver dysfunction. Nutritional shortcomings, for instance imbalance of essential fatty acids, are common among people who suffer from itchy skin. Often the cause is in the environment in the form of washing powder or bubble bath. If the itch persists in spite of the measures described below, consult a health professional.

Treatment options

- Apply calendula ointment daily if your skin looks dry (for precautions see page 114). *Adults and children over 2 years old:* 1-2 times a day.

- Add calendula infused oil to your bath (for precautions see page 114). *Adults and children over 2 years old:* 10ml, once a day, until the skin improves.

- Add thyme or calendula to your bath, either as a tincture or as a strong tea (for precautions see page 114). *Adults and children over 2 years old:* you need to add enough herbs so that the bath water becomes slightly yellow in colour, roughly about 40ml of tincture or ½ litre of infusion. Do this once a day for a week.

NAPPY RASH

Warning: Be careful if your baby suffers from eczema – occasionally herbal preparations can make it worse.

Nappy rash occurs when the baby's skin becomes irritated by its own urine or faeces. Keeping the nappy area well covered in a special protective cream will prevent the problem from occurring in the first place. Sometimes nappy rash is also caused by baby wipes or other baby skin products, which may contain irritating ingredients.

Treatment options

- Apply calendula cream to the nappy area, and leave the baby without a nappy for a while after the application. For precautions see page 114. *Dosage:* 1-2 times a day.

- Add some calendula **tea** to the baby bath to promote healing. *Dosage:* 1 cup of infusion per bath, 2-3 days in a row. For precautions see page 114.

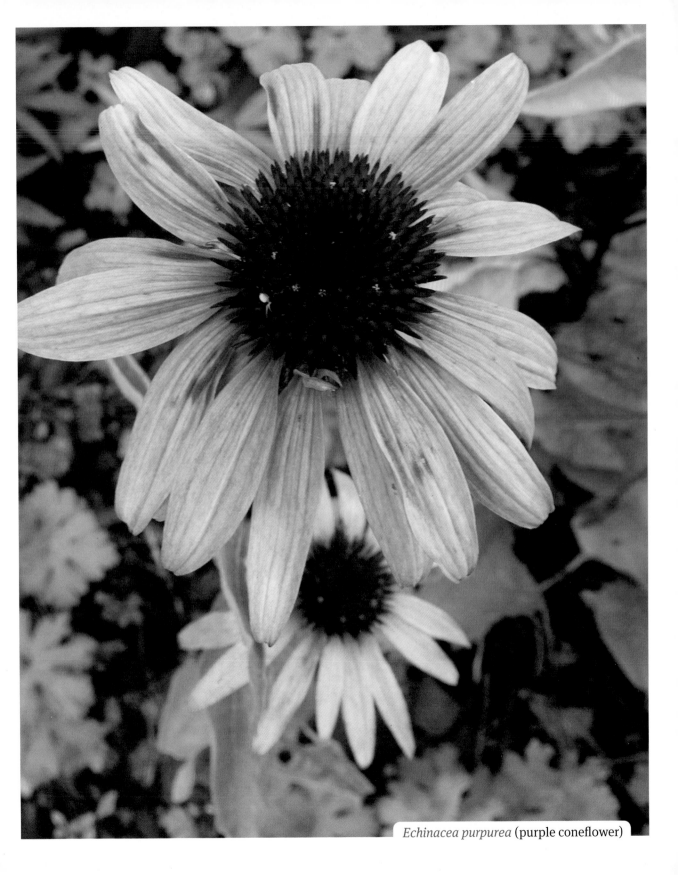

Echinacea purpurea (purple coneflower)

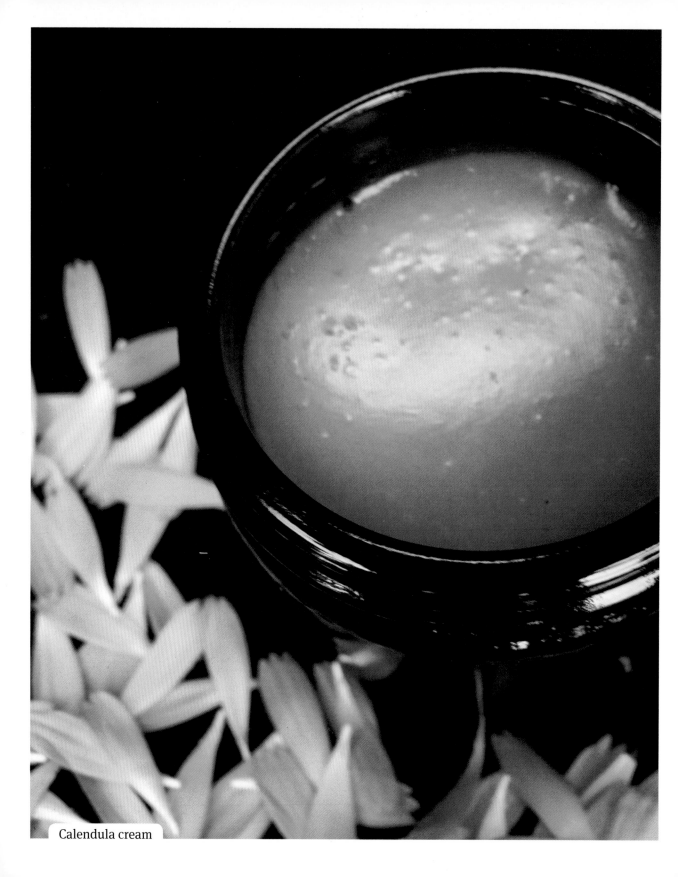

Calendula cream

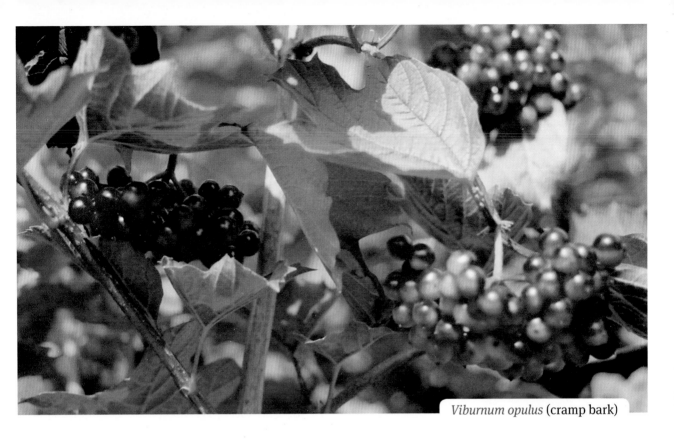

Viburnum opulus (cramp bark)

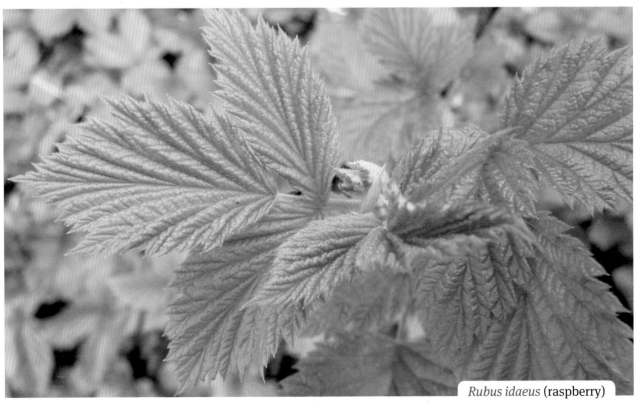

Rubus idaeus (raspberry)

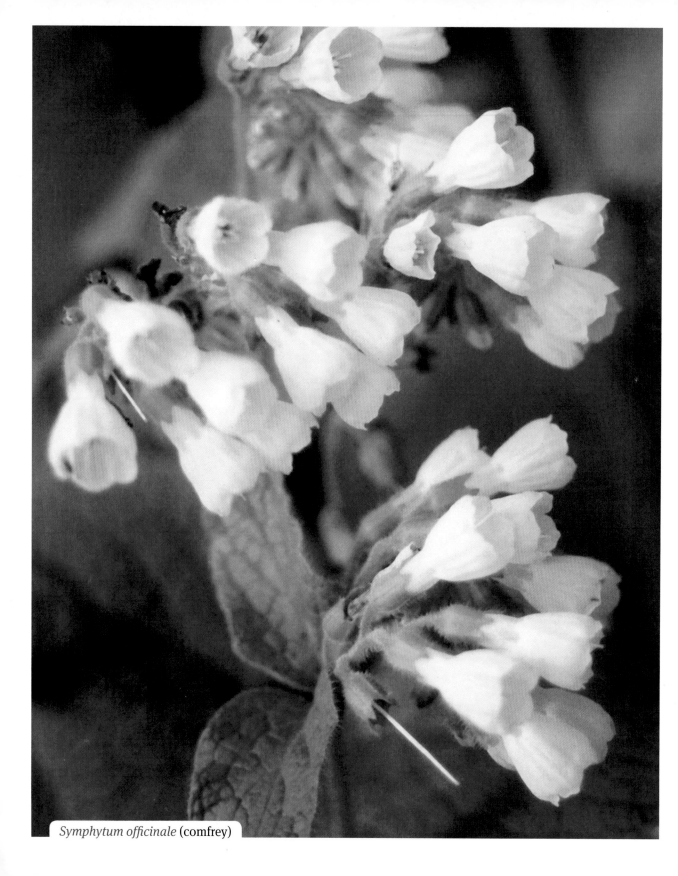

Symphytum officinale (comfrey)

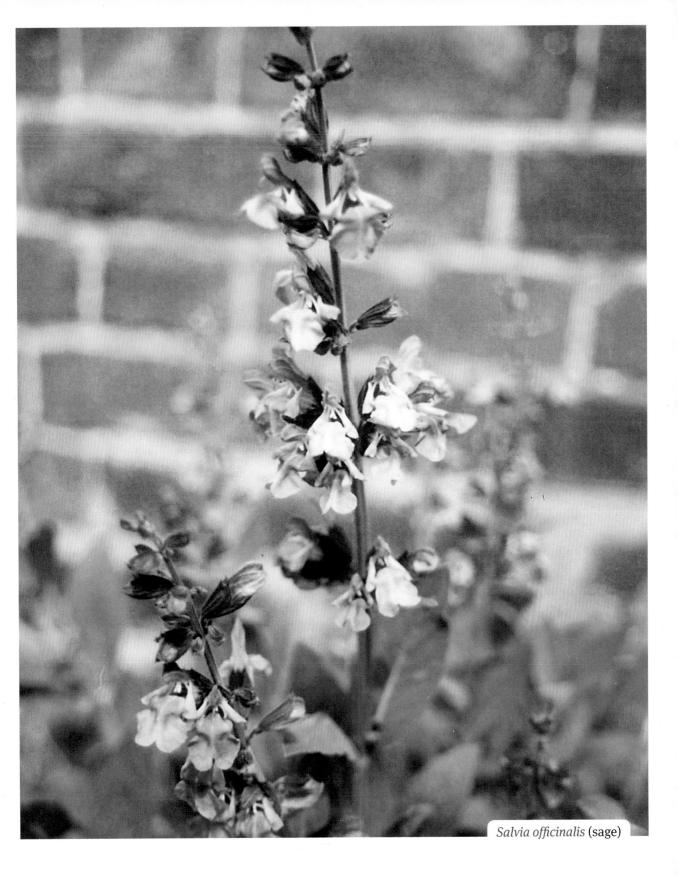

Salvia officinalis (sage)

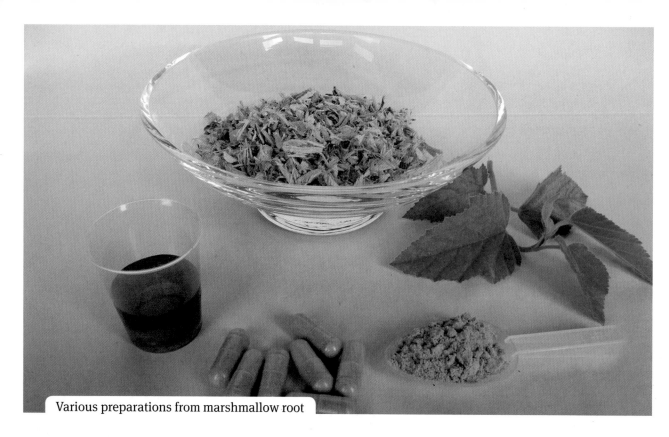

Various preparations from marshmallow root

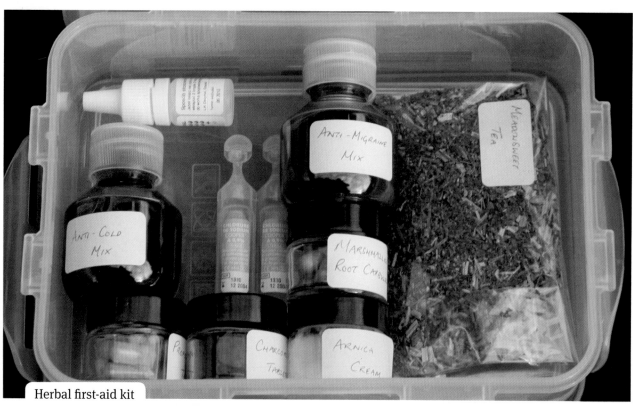

Herbal first-aid kit

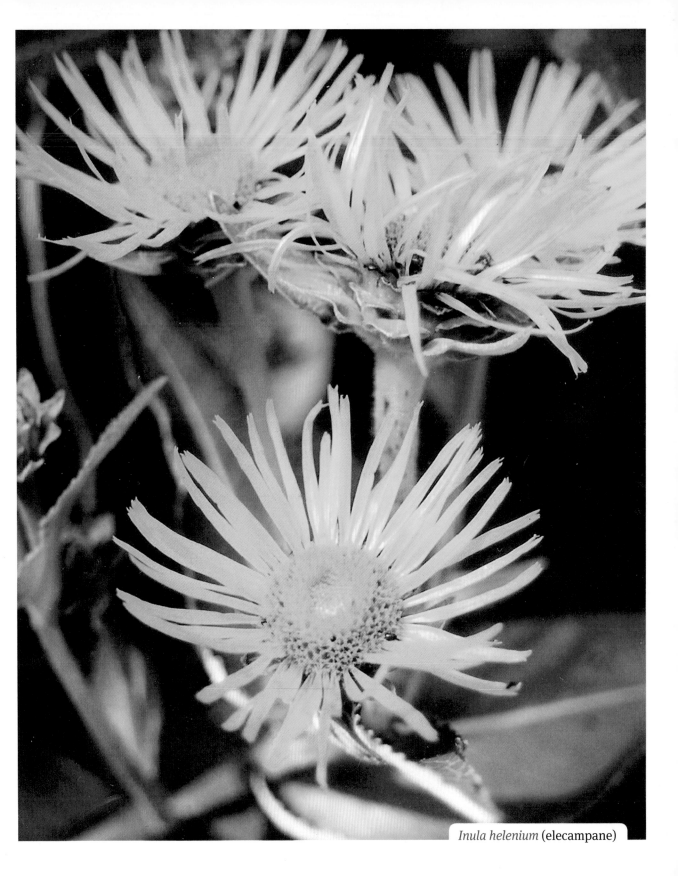

Inula helenium (elecampane)

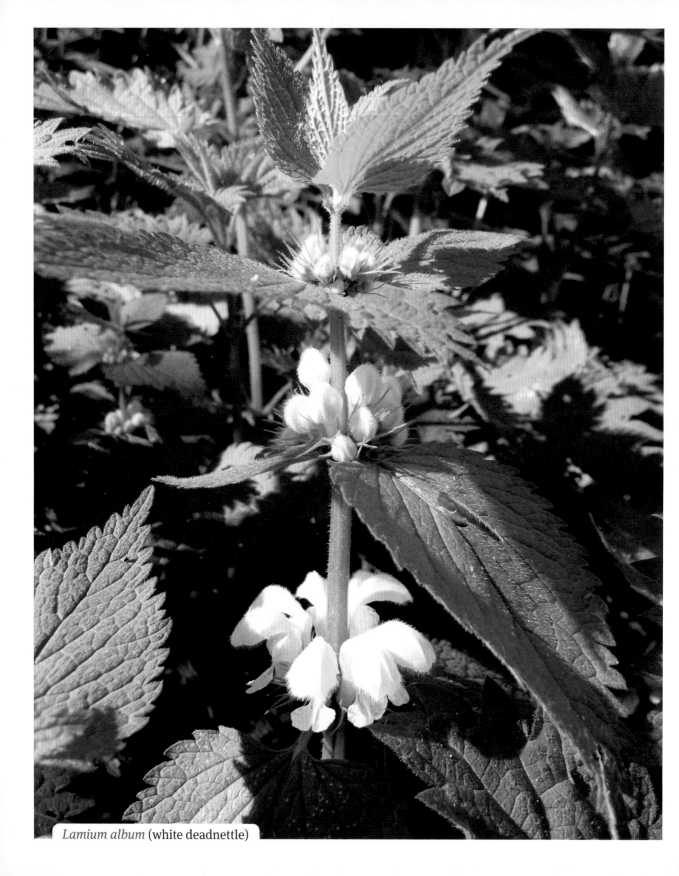

Lamium album (white deadnettle)

PSORIASIS

Practitioner treatment is recommended for this condition.

Psoriasis is a complex disease, and the treatments for it are exceptionally diverse and individual – in short, there is no universal treatment. Dietary factors and lifestyle play a large role and often need to be adjusted. The measures below will benefit some people, but most will need a unique treatment tailored to their own specific circumstances. The treatment for psoriasis is long term – at least a year.

Treatment options

- Take mountain grape tincture (for precautions see page 117). *Adults:* 1-2.5ml, 1-3 times a day, tincture strength 1:2.

- Apply a cream for psoriasis with St John's wort infused oil – see box below.

- Take the mix for skin disorders – see box on the right.

Children (2-16 years old): adjust the internal adult dose downwards, depending on the age of the child – see Chapter 6.

CREAM FOR PSORIASIS
Ingredients
- 20g calendula or comfrey cream
- 5ml St John's wort infused oil

To make
- Mix well.
- Transfer to a clean, dark glass jar making sure that there are no air pockets left.
- Store for up to 12 months.

Adults and children over 2 years: apply to the affected areas twice a day.

MIX FOR SKIN DISORDERS
Ingredients
- 20ml yellow dock (tincture strength 1:5) (for precautions see page 119)
- 20ml red clover (tincture strength 1:2)
- 20ml mountain grape (tincture strength 1:2) (for precautions see page 117)
- 40ml ribwort plantain (tincture strength 1:2)

To make
- Mix ingredients together.
- Pour into a clean, dark glass bottle.
- Label with the contents and the date.
- Store at room temperature for up to a year.

Adult dose: 5ml diluted with some water, 2-3 times a day.

PUFFY EYES / TIRED EYES

Swollen eyelids or swollen areas underneath the eyes can be a sign of tiredness, allergy or water retention. If it happens regularly you should consult a health professional to find out what the underlying cause is. But if it is a one-off occurrence, the measures below will bring rapid improvement. The same measures can be used for tired eyes that feel uncomfortable due to lack of sleep or over-work. It is best to lie down for these treatments so that you can close your eyes and relax.

Treatment options

Both these options are suitable for children over 2 years old.

- Make a compress from ordinary, strong, black tea, and apply for 10 minutes. Use cotton wool soaked in freshly brewed warm tea, squeeze gently and apply as eye compresses (you don't want the compresses to dribble but you don't want to squeeze them too much either, otherwise they will be too dry to have an effect). You may need to re-soak the cotton wool pads if they get cold. This is surprisingly effective and a good option for people allergic to calendula or chamomile.

- Make a compress from strong chamomile tea and apply for 10 minutes, as above, as long as you know that you do not react adversely to chamomile (for precautions see page 114).

SKIN RASH

Skin rash can be a reaction to heat, cosmetics or contact with plants and many other substances. You should see a health professional for a proper diagnosis. It is important to get the right diagnosis as many skin problems may look the same to the untrained eye: for instance, some forms of eczema look like fungal infections or heat rash, and vice versa. Because treatment will depend on the under-lying cause, the measures below are of a rather general nature: they calm down the inflamma-tion and stimulate the natural healing processes.

Treatment options

- Apply calendula ointment until the rash disappears (discontinue this treatment if the rash becomes worse). For precautions see page 114. *Adults and children over 2 years old:* 1-2 times a day.

- Apply a ribwort plantain poultice or compress; you can use fresh or dry herbs. This is an extremely soothing treatment

that can be applied even to a rash that oozes fluid, such as weeping eczema. See pages 24 and 23 for instructions on how to prepare and apply a poultice or compress. *Adults and children over 2 years old:* apply 1-2 times a day for 15 minutes each time.

SKIN INFECTION

Warning: Urgent medical help must be sought in some circumstances – see below.

A skin infection usually follows some kind of injury: a cut, a scratch, a prick or a sting. Normally bacteria cannot penetrate the intact skin, and only when it is broken do the bacteria gain access to the deeper layers. The signs of infection are: swelling around the point of entry, redness and tenderness. You may have a raised temperature. You must watch out for a red streak developing away from the infected area: this indicates that the infection is spreading through your blood and there is a high risk of septicaemia (blood infection). If you notice this, seek medical help urgently. However, most local infections are easy to treat with herbs: I recommend the combined treatment of both an external and an internal antibacterial remedy.

Treatment options

- Eat raw garlic daily until the infection goes (for precautions see page 96). *Adults:* 1 crushed clove of garlic mixed with a teaspoon of honey, 2-3 times a day.

- You can fix a slice of garlic to the area with a plaster, but don't leave it in place for more than 2-3 hours or you may end up with a local skin reaction that looks a bit like a burn. For children you can rub the infected area with a sliced clove of garlic 1-2 times a day.

- Take propolis tincture (for precautions see page 99). *Adults:* 1-2ml, 2-3 times a day, tincture strength 1:10; or propolis capsules that are equivalent to 2-3g of propolis a day.
- Apply strongly antiseptic cream for skin infections – see box below.

Children (3-16 years old): adjust the internal adult dose downwards, depending on the age of the child – see Chapter 6.

CREAM FOR SKIN INFECTIONS

Ingredients
- 50g calendula cream (for precautions see page 114)
- 10ml echinacea tincture (for precautions see page 115)
- 10 drops of thyme essential oil (for precautions see page 115)
- 10 drops of tea tree essential oil (for precautions see page 118)

To make
- Mix well.
- Transfer to a clean, dark glass jar, making sure that there are no air pockets left.
- Store for up to 12 months.

Adults and children over 3 years old: Apply a good layer to the infected area and cover with non-absorbent dressing (you want the ointment to be absorbed into the skin, not into the dressing); change every 3-4 hours until the redness and swelling are visibly reduced and there is no tenderness.

SPLINTERS

Small splinters that cannot be pulled out with tweezers can be drawn out with a paste made from herbal powder.

Treatment options

Both these options are suitable for children over 2 years old and in pregnancy.

- Mix a teaspoon of marshmallow root powder with a little warm water to form a thick paste. Apply the paste to the area where the splinter is, cover with a small square of plastic or Clingfilm and then with sticking plaster. Keep the dressing on for an hour or so. When you remove the dressing there is usually no sign of the splinter but the skin may look 'puckered' for a while.

- If the area around the splinter is inflamed, add 1 drop of thyme or tea tree essential oil to the paste and proceed as above.

STYE

Practitioner treatment is recommended for this condition.

A stye is a painful infection that affects the eyelid margins. It usually indicates poor immune function, exhaustion and dietary deficiencies. The contributing factors need to be looked at in addition to the external treatment.

Treatment options

- Apply a small amount of calendula ointment directly to the stye until the symptoms disappear completely. Use a cotton bud for precise application and make sure the ointment does not get into the eye. For precautions see page 114. *Adults and children over 2 years old:* apply 3-5 times a day.

- Apply a calendula compress 2 times a day to the affected eye (follow the instructions for eyebright compress, page 124). For precautions see page 114.

- Take eyebright tincture for a month. *Adults:* 1-2ml diluted with some water, 2 times a day, tincture strength 1:2.

Children (2-16 years old): adjust the internal adult dose downwards, depending on the age of the child – see Chapter 6.

- Apply a small amount of propolis cream directly to the stye until the symptoms disappear completely – see box below.

PROPOLIS CREAM
Ingredients
- 50g calendula or comfrey cream (for precautions see page 114)
- 5ml propolis tincture (for precautions see page 99)

To make
- Mix well.
- Transfer to a clean, dark glass jar, making sure that there are no air pockets left.
- Store for up to 12 months.

Adults and children over 2 years old: apply to the stye 3-5 times a day.

SUNBURN

Sunburn can vary from a mild pinkness of the skin to a flaming red skin covered in blisters. If your sunburn is severe do not use tinctures externally, as even a tiny amount of alcohol will sting. Calendula provides the best treatment I have ever come across, the calendula compress being immediately cooling and reducing the pain. Apply a cool but not ice-cold treatment.

Treatment options

All these options are suitable for children over 2 years old.

- Have a lukewarm bath with added calendula tincture or strong calendula tea; add enough to make the bath water yellowish in colour. Soak for 10-15 minutes. For precautions see page 114.

- Apply cooled calendula tea directly to the skin with a sponge or cotton wool; gently dab every hour until there is noticeable relief. For precautions see page 114.

- Apply a cool calendula tea compress (see page 23 for instructions on making a compress) For precautions see page 114. *Dosage:* this can be done repeatedly until relief is felt; usually 2 or 3 applications are sufficient, but more may be necessary for a really bad sunburn.

- Apply calendula ointment/cream – this is best done after one of the above cooling treatments; the calendula ointment prevents the skin peeling later on, as well as providing a soothing effect. For precautions see page 114. *Dosage:* one generous application is usually sufficient.

- Apply thyme tincture diluted with cold

water as a gentle wipe; this is suitable for minor sunburns. *Dosage:* 20ml of tincture per cup of cool water; apply hourly 2-3 times.

Warts / verrucas

You need to be persistent in treating warts, as they often take a long time to disappear.

Warts that don't diminish with the treatments described below, or widespread warts, may require an internal treatment.

Treatment options

- Apply a sliver of fresh garlic directly to the wart and hold it in place with a plaster for 2-3 hours (warning: garlic may sting and cause a temporary skin rash around the wart). This is a one-off treatment, and I do not recommend this treatment for small children under 6 years old.

- Apply thuja tincture to the wart for a few weeks. *Adults and children over 2 years old:* apply one drop in the morning and evening until the wart is gone.

- Apply fresh dandelion sap directly to the wart for a few weeks. This treatment works best in the spring when dandelions are flowering. *Adults and children over 2 years old:* break a flowering stem and apply the fresh white juice to the wart 2-4 times a day.

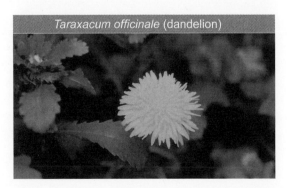
Taraxacum officinale (dandelion)

WHEN AND WHY YOU SHOULD SEE A PROFESSIONAL MEDICAL HERBALIST

- Widespread eczema: this requires a comprehensive review of diet and lifestyle as well as individual internal treatment.

- Psoriasis: the treatment varies from person to person enormously and may take up to a year.

- Acne rosacea: this is a complex condition that needs treatment of the circulatory system as well as the skin; it requires long-term medicating with herbs.

- Molluscum contagiosum: although this viral infection will resolve itself eventually, herbal treatment can considerably speed the recovery time.

- Multiple warts: these usually require a combination of external and internal treatment.

- Fungal infection of the nails that cannot be eradicated: persistent fungal infection of the nails often requires an internal treatment as well as a combination of external remedies that can be rotated.

- Urticaria (hives): this condition is allergic in nature and therefore needs careful treatment; attending to lifestyle and stress factors is often necessary.

- Skin ulcer: a specialised treatment is required both internally and externally; you may need supervision on a daily or weekly basis to make sure that a particular treatment option is working.

THE FOLLOWING SYMPTOMS WARRANT SEEING A HEALTH PROFESSIONAL WITHOUT DELAY

- Eye infection (conjunctivitis).

- Infected cut or wound that won't heal, especially if there is a lot of redness around the area and a red streak developing on the skin in the direction of blood circulation (this indicates the spread of the local infection, and there is a danger of septicaemia).

- Sudden, patchy loss of hair.

- Impetigo – skin infection that produces yellow crusting and spreads quickly.

- Fungal infection of the scalp.

- Widespread fungal infection of the skin.

- Any unusual and persistent skin rash.

- Any skin lump that is tender, or does not go away, or becomes enlarged.

- Any mole that changes appearance and becomes enlarged or ulcerates.

Chapter 16
The urinary and reproductive systems

Although the urinary and reproductive systems are two independent physiological systems, they are closely connected through their proximity in the anatomy and the influence of sex hormones.

THE URINARY SYSTEM

The urinary system in males and females is essentially the same and consists of the kidneys, ureter, bladder and urethra. The latter is much shorter in women than in men, which explains to an extent the higher prevalence of urinary tract infections in females. Infections of the urinary tract, if limited to its lower parts (urethra and bladder), can be successfully treated at home, but if they are persistent you must consult your GP or a medical herbalist to make sure that the infection doesn't spread to the kidneys, which is potentially dangerous.

FEMALE REPRODUCTIVE SYSTEM

The reproductive system in women includes the vagina, uterus and ovaries, and it is governed by a complicated interplay of sex hormones. Only mild hormonal irregularities are suitable for self-treatment, but other common ailments of the female reproductive system yield themselves to home treatment easily. Some problems related to pregnancy (nausea, reflux) are discussed in other sections (see pages 63 and 62), while more serious problems should be treated under the supervision of a medical herbalist.

MALE REPRODUCTIVE SYSTEM

The reproductive system in men includes the penis, testicles and prostate gland. The disorders of the male reproductive system can also have their root cause in the dysfunction of hormonal control, but often stem from lifestyle, circulatory disease or psychological issues. Only a small selection of such problems can be successfully treated at home.

HERB SELECTION IN THIS CHAPTER

It is difficult to pick a small selection of herbs for the variety of medical problems that can affect the urinary and reproductive systems. The main reason is that such herbs often have a very narrow spectrum of action: for instance, saw palmetto is specifically used to treat prostate problems. It may not be practical to store many of the herbs needed to effectively treat these systems unless you already use some of these herbs for other problems. The selection below, which is perhaps larger than that for any other system, will cover quite a few problems, but for many ailments of the urinary and reproductive systems you will need additional herbs.

MUST-HAVE HERBS

The herbs in this section are arranged in order of usefulness.

MARSHMALLOW LEAF

Uses
You can use marshmallow leaf to make a very soothing drink if you have cystitis or urethritis. Marshmallow leaf provides really quick relief from the pain and stinging sensation in the urethra.

How to take
As a tea. Start drinking it as soon as you develop symptoms of cystitis or urethritis. It is best to drink this tea warm and let it brew for a long time to allow the release of the mucilage (the anti-irritant constituent of the plant) from the leaves. You can infuse a large amount of the herb (10 teaspoonsful) in one go in a cafetière or a teapot and then drink 3-5 portions throughout the day, mixing each portion with a bit of hot water.

Dosage
Adults: 3-5 large cups a day.
Children (2-16 years old): adjust the adult dose downwards, depending on the age of the child – see Chapter 6.

CRAMP BARK

Uses
Cramp bark is a muscular relaxant, therefore suitable for alleviating cramping period pain.

How to take
Take it as and when needed, in tincture form.

Dosage
Adults: if you experience period cramps take 2ml diluted with some water 3 times a day, tincture strength 1:2, for 1-2 days.
Teenagers (11-16 years old): adjust the adult dose downwards, depending on the age of the child – see Chapter 6.

COUCH GRASS

Uses
Couch grass is mildly diuretic and soothes irritation in the urinary tract. It is suitable for those situations when passing urine causes pain or a burning sensation (cystitis, urethritis) or when there is a general inflammation of particular parts of the urinary tract (prostatitis, kidney stones).

Combinations
Couch grass combines well with urinary antiseptics such as thyme, celery seed and mountain grape, and with other anti-irritants, for instance marshmallow leaf.

How to take
Couch grass can be taken as a tea or as a tincture.

Dosage
Adults: 1-2ml diluted with some water 3 times a day, tincture strength 1:1; or 3-4 cups of tea a day.
Children (2-16 years old): adjust the adult dose downwards, depending on the age of the child – see Chapter 6.

ECHINACEA (PURPLE CONEFLOWER)

Caution needed if allergic to plants of the *Compositae* family.

Uses

As a general immune system modulator echinacea can be taken to help with any infection, therefore it is a useful supplement if you have repeated bouts of cystitis or thrush.

How to take

Take it for at least a month to boost your immune system after the worst of your infection is over.

Dosage

Adults: 1-2ml diluted with some water, 2-3 times a day, tincture strength 1:5.
Children (2-16 years old): adjust the adult dose downwards, depending on the age of the child – see Chapter 6.

THYME

Uses

Thyme works as an antiseptic for the urinary system, therefore it is used for urinary tract infections. It is also useful for thrush.

How to take

To treat cystitis, take thyme as tincture until the symptoms completely disappear. It is best to drink marshmallow leaf tea at the same time. For thrush, take thyme tincture as well as echinacea tincture.

Dosage

Adults: 0.7-1.5ml diluted with some water, 2-3 times a day, tincture strength 1:2.
Children (2-16 years old): adjust the adult dose downwards, depending on the age of the child – see Chapter 6.

VALERIAN

Uses

Valerian is a very useful addition for some problems of the urinary and reproductive systems when there is a connection to stress – for instance, if you feel marked tension and irritability before periods, if you cannot sleep because of hot flushes or if you suffer from an urgency to pass water whenever you feel nervous.

How to take

You can take valerian at a long-term dosage if the problem is long-term, or as a larger one-off dose if the problem is occasional in nature.

Dosage

Adults (long-term): 0.3-1ml diluted with some water, 1-3 times a day, tincture strength 1:1.
Adults (one-off dose): 5ml diluted with some water, 1-2 times a day, tincture strength 1:1.
Children (2-16 years old): adjust the adult dose downwards, depending on the age of the child – see Chapter 6.

YARROW

Warning: Do not take if pregnant.
Caution needed if allergic to plants of the *Compositae* family.

Uses

This herb can be used for periods that are irregular, too heavy or too light. It is also good if your digestion is not right around the time of your period.

Combinations

It combines well with herbs such as valerian, chamomile or cramp bark to reduce period pain.

How to take

Take it as a tea or tincture.

Dosage

Adults: 1-2 cups a day or 0.7-2ml, 1-3 times a day, tincture strength 1:2.

Teenagers (11-16 years old): adjust the adult dose downwards, depending on the age of the teenager – see Chapter 6.

SAW PALMETTO

Warning: Not suitable for children.

Caution: Possibility of a temporary gastric upset.

Caution needed if taking warfarin.

Uses

This herb is specific for prostate problems but it can also be used in other inflammatory disorders of the male genito-urinary tract such as urethritis or orchitis.

Sometimes it can cause an upset stomach or upset bowels, in which case it needs to be combined with herbs that are anti-irritant to the digestive system (for instance marshmallow root, see page 48).

How to take

It can be taken in tincture, capsule or tablet form.

Dosage

Adults only: 1-3ml, 2-3 times a day, tincture strength 1:2; or the equivalent of 2.2-3.2g of dry herb a day as tablets or capsules.

OPTIONAL HERBS

SELECTION OF DIURETIC TEAS

Many herbs discussed in previous chapters have diuretic properties, and as such can be used whenever it is desirable to increase the volume of urine – for instance, during a bout of cystitis or urethritis. It is preferable to have diuretic herbs in a tea form, but a tincture diluted with a cupful of warm water will work just as well. You can choose from the following herbs: marshmallow leaf, celery seed (for precautions see page 139), birch, shepherd's purse (for precautions see page 140), dandelion leaf, lime tree flower or nettle leaf.

BLACK COHOSH

Warning: If you develop any abdominal discomfort, discontinue taking this herb and consult a health professional. Do not take if you have a history of liver problems, or if you take any medication (conventional or herbal, including over-the-counter products) or if you are pregnant.

Not suitable for children.

I strongly recommend that you get this herb prescribed by a medical herbalist.

Uses
Black cohosh is often recommended to menopausal women for a range of problems associated with the menopause (hot flushes or night sweats, mood swings, joint pain or low libido). Although it can be effective on its own, better results are usually achieved when combined with other herbs in an individual prescription.

How to take
As a tincture. I recommend starting this herb in small doses, as some people react to larger doses with a severe headache. If you are fine with a low dosage you can gradually increase the dose.

Dosage
Adults (over 16 years old): initially 5 drops diluted with some water 2-3 times a day, tincture strength 1:5, gradually increasing to 10 drops diluted with some water 2-3 times a day.

CELERY SEED

> **Caution needed** if you have a kidney disorder or when breastfeeding.

Uses
Celery seed is most useful for infections of the urinary tract, as it is an antiseptic for this part of the body.

How to take
As a tincture. It combines well with couch grass (see page 136).

Dosage
Adults: 1.5-3ml diluted with some water, 1-3 times a day, tincture strength 1:2.

Children (2-16 years old): adjust the adult dose downwards, depending on the age of the child – see Chapter 6.

DAMIANA

> **Warning:** Not suitable for children.
> **Caution needed** if prone to extreme anxiety.

Uses
Damiana is considered a tonic for both the male and female reproductive systems, and can therefore be used in a number of circumstances when these do not function optimally. It seems to possess a mild aphrodisiac action as well as providing a general sense of well-being.

How to take
As a tincture.

Dosage
Adults: 1-2ml diluted with some water, 1-3 times a day, tincture strength 1:2.

SAGE

> **Warning:** Do not take internally when pregnant or breastfeeding.
> Do not take continually for long periods of time.
> Not suitable for children.

Uses
Sage preparations inhibit sweating and hence come in useful for hot flushes. It is best to combine this herb with other herbs for menopausal symptoms.

How to take

You should not take sage continually, so have a 2-week break every 4 weeks or so.

Dosage

Adults only: 0.7-1.4ml diluted with some water, 2-3 times a day, tincture strength 1:2.

SHEPHERD'S PURSE

Caution needed if pregnant and when breastfeeding.

Uses

This herb can be used to decrease the amount of bleeding during a heavy period, but a large dose is needed to achieve this effect. Shepherd's purse can also improve the tone of the uterus muscle and can help with a partial uterine prolapse.

How to take

As a tincture or tea.

Dosage

Adults (heavy periods): 10ml diluted with some water, 3-4 times a day, tincture strength 1:2, for 1-2 days only.
Adults (uterine tone): 2-3 cups of tea a day, or 1-2ml diluted with some water, 3 times a day, tincture strength 1:2, until symptoms improve.
Teenagers (11-16 years old): adjust the adult dose downwards, depending on the age of the child – see Chapter 6.

WHITE DEAD NETTLE

Uses

This herb is used specifically for excessive vaginal discharge. It provides a useful addition to the treatment of thrush or other infections of the female reproductive tract.

Combinations

It combines well with thyme and calendula, either as a tincture or tea.

How to take

As a tincture or tea.
Adults: 1-2 cups of tea a day; or 2ml diluted with some water, 2-3 times a day, tincture strength 1:5.
Teenagers (11-16 years old): adjust the adult dose downwards, depending on the age of the child – see Chapter 6.

WILD YAM

Uses

Wild yam is one of the main herbs used for the treatment of menopausal problems. It is especially useful if the sufferer also has rheumatic or arthritic symptoms.

Combine it with other herbs depending on the particular array of menopausal symptoms (see the Menopause entry, page 145).

How to take

As a tincture.

Dosage

Adults: 1-2ml diluted with some water, 2-3 times a day, tincture strength 1:2.

SPECIFIC AILMENTS OF THE URINARY AND REPRODUCTIVE SYSTEMS & HERBS THAT CAN HELP

BEDWETTING (CHILDREN)

This problem normally resolves itself as the child grows up, but a gentle herbal support may help with the natural maturing of the brain–bladder alarm system. Sometimes emotional issues are involved, in which case you should seek professional help.

Treatment options

- Cramp bark tincture. *Children (3-7 years old):* 7 drops diluted in water/juice, 2 times a day, tincture strength 1:2.

- Marshmallow leaf tea. *Children (3-7 years old):* a quarter of a cup 2 times a day.

BENIGN PROSTATIC ENLARGEMENT (HYPERTROPHY)

Practitioner treatment is recommended for this condition.

This condition must be diagnosed by a GP as the symptoms are identical to those of a prostate malignancy. Herbs can bring relief from needing to pass water frequently, especially at night. Men with prostatic enlargement are prone to cystitis and urine retention, both of which can be successfully treated with herbs without the need for antibiotics.

Treatment options

- Take saw palmetto tincture on a regular basis (for precautions see page 138). *Adults only:* 1-3ml diluted with some water, 2-3 times a day, tincture strength 1:2.

- Drink marshmallow leaf and nettle leaf tea – see box below – on a daily basis to prevent cystitis.

TEA FOR PREVENTING CYSTITIS

Ingredients
- 50g dry marshmallow leaf
- 25g dry nettle leaf

To make
- Mix herbs thoroughly.
- Infuse 2 teaspoonsful of the mix in a cupful of freshly boiled water for 10 minutes. Strain and drink warm.

Adult dose: 1 cup a day for 3-12 months.

CYSTITIS AND URETHRITIS

Practitioner treatment is recommended for recurrent episodes.

Cystitis is an infection of the bladder, and it is as common as urethritis, which is an infection of the urethra (the narrow passage connecting the bladder to the outside of the body). If your symptoms consist of a burning sensation on passing urine, an urgency to pass water, and you need to pass water very often, you are most likely to be suffering from urethritis. If, on top of the above, you develop a pain above your pubic bone, become feverish and your urine becomes cloudy and smelly, you are most likely suffering from cystitis. Apart from taking the herbs described below, it is important to drink a lot of water (1 litre a day) to dilute the urine, as this will reduce the stinging and flush out the bacteria. Another common measure is to drink cranberry juice, preferably diluted and unsweetened, although this is only effective for some bacteria that can infect the urinary tract. You can also speed recovery by eating lots of parsley and celery, avoiding hot spices and alcohol, and taking yourself to bed with a hot water bottle.

Remember that if your infection does not clear within a couple of days you must see a health practitioner, as there is always the potential of the infection spreading to the kidneys. If you notice that there is a link between your cystitis and sexual activity, be fastidious about your and your partner's hygiene, and empty your bladder both before and after sex.

Treatment options

The treatment for both cystitis and urethritis is the same.

- Drink marshmallow leaf tea to soothe the pain and the irritation. *Adults:* 3-5 cups a day.

- Drink any of the diuretic teas listed in the optional herbs section, page 138. *Adults:* 1 cup a day if you are already drinking marshmallow tea, otherwise 3 cups a day.

- Take thyme tincture for its antiseptic properties (if you are not taking the mix for cystitis, see right). *Adults:* 0.7-1.5ml diluted with some water, 1-3 times a day, tincture strength 1:2.

- Take echinacea tincture if you suffer recurrent episodes (for precautions see page 137). *Adults:* 1-2ml diluted with some

water, 2-3 times a day for a month, tincture strength 1:5.

- Take the mix for cystitis and urethritis – see box below.

Children (2-16 years old): adjust the adult dose downwards, depending on the age of the child – see Chapter 6.

MIX FOR URETHRITIS AND CYSTITIS

Ingredients
- 20ml thyme (tincture strength 1:2)
- 20ml celery seed (tincture strength 1:2) (for precautions see page 139)
- 20ml couch grass (tincture strength 1:1)
- 40ml marshmallow leaf (tincture strength 1:2)

To make
- Mix ingredients together.
- Pour into a clean, dark glass bottle.
- Label with the contents and the date.
- Store at room temperature for up to a year.

Adult dose: 10ml diluted with some water for the first dose, then 5ml diluted with some water twice more that day and then 3 times a day until the symptoms are gone, and for one further day after the symptoms are gone.

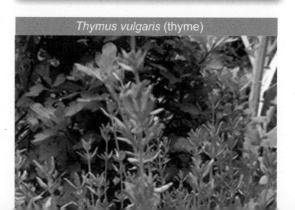

Thymus vulgaris (thyme)

ERECTILE DYSFUNCTION

> Practitioner treatment is recommended for this condition.

Erectile dysfunction can be a complex ailment, with diverse causes such as having diabetes, taking particular medication, drinking too much alcohol or having psychological problems. You need to address the causes, and often the primary treatment may be long. The measures below can provide supportive treatment only.

Treatment options

- Improve your circulation with hawthorn and blueberries (see Chapter 10, pages 37 and 36, for more information).

- Take relaxing herbs if anxiety is an issue (see Chapter 13, page 86).

HOT FLUSHES

> Practitioner treatment is recommended for this condition.

Hot flushes are often experienced by women around the menopause, most often after their periods have stopped. Many herbs and supplements can be useful, although the choice of appropriate herbs depends on where you are in terms of your menopause. For instance, if you still have your periods, chaste tree can be helpful, but if you have stopped having periods or have had a total hysterectomy, chaste tree would be a waste of time.

A proper diet can make a big difference: for example, eating less meat and more soya products. Supplements of vitamin E can be helpful to some women (400-500iu a day). If hot flushes are really bad you will need a complex prescription to balance your female sex hormones as well as other hormones, especially thyroid hormones. If your hot flushes are caused by side effects of your medication you should consult a practitioner before taking any herbs.

Treatment options

- Take black cohosh tincture, but remember not to combine black cohosh with any conventional or herbal over-the-counter medicines. For precautions see page 138. *Adults:* 5 drops diluted with some water, 2-3 times a day, tincture strength 1:2, increasing to 10 drops, 2-3 times a day if no side effects are experienced.

- Take sage tincture – but take a 2-week break from this herb every 4 weeks if you take a large dose. For precautions see page 102. *Adults:* 0.7-1.4ml diluted with some water, 2-3 times a day, tincture strength 1:2.

- Take wild yam tincture. *Adults:* 1-2ml diluted with some water, 2-3 times a day, tincture strength 1:2.

- Take hawthorn flower tincture. For precautions see page 37. *Adults:* 1-2ml diluted with some water, 1-3 times a day, tincture strength 1:2.

- Take St John's wort tincture if the menopausal symptoms bring you down. *Adults:* 0.6-2ml diluted with some water, 2-3 times a day, tincture strength 1:2. For precautions see page 85.

- Take the mix for hot flushes – see box overleaf – but take it instead of, not as well as, the above herbs.

MIX FOR HOT FLUSHES

Ingredients

- 5ml black cohosh (tincture strength 1:2) (for precautions see page 138)
- 20ml sage (tincture strength 1:2) (for precautions see page 102)
- 35ml wild yam (tincture strength 1:2)
- 20ml hawthorn flowers (tincture strength 1:2) (for precautions see page 37)
- 20ml St John's wort (tincture strength 1:2) (for precautions see page 85)

To make

- Mix ingredients together.
- Pour into a clean, dark glass bottle.
- Label with the contents and the date.
- Store at room temperature for up to a year.

Adults only: 5ml diluted with some water, 2-3 times a day.

INCONTINENCE

Practitioner treatment is recommended for this condition.

Inability to hold urine can affect both males and females, and can be a result of many factors, e.g. stress, infection, weakness of the pelvic floor muscles, urine retention, post-surgery inflammation, etc. With such a variety of causes the core treatment will vary from person to person and should be prescribed by a medical herbalist. The measures below are therefore meant to provide only a supportive treatment to the main prescribed treatment.

Treatment options

- Drink marshmallow leaf tea daily to reduce any irritation that leads to an urgent need to pass urine. *Adults:* 2-3 cups a day.

- Drink shepherd's purse tea as a gentle diuretic that helps with urine retention. For precautions see page 140. *Adults :* 2-3 cups a day.

Children (2-16 years old): adjust the adult dose downwards, depending on the age of the child – see Chapter 6.

LIBIDO, LOW

This is a surprisingly common problem in both sexes, which usually has its root causes in overwork, emotional complaints and lifestyle issues; occasionally unbalanced hormones can be blamed. There is more information on improving sex drive in Chapter 19.

Treatment options

- Take damiana tincture (for precautions see page 139). *Adults:* 1-2ml diluted with some water, 1-3 times a day, tincture strength 1:2.

- Take Korean ginseng as a general tonic for the whole body, which also improves the sex drive. For precautions see page 153. *Adults:* 300-500mg a day (tablet form) or 0.5-2.5ml diluted with some water, 1-2 times a day, tincture strength 1:2.

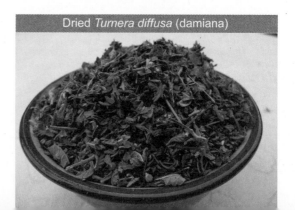
Dried *Turnera diffusa* (damiana)

Menopausal problems

Practitioner treatment is recommended for this condition.

The menopause can bring an array of health problems: hot flushes, mood swings, low libido, discomfort during sex and joint aches. Each woman will have an individual set of symptoms that will vary in severity. And each woman will need an individual prescription, which may need to be adjusted as the symptoms improve. Therefore the two prescriptions here will suit only a proportion of women and should be customised to treat your unique set of symptoms.

MIX FOR MENOPAUSAL SYMPTOMS (MAIN PROBLEM: HOT FLUSHES)

Ingredients
- 20ml sage (tincture strength 1:2) (for precautions see page 102)
- 20ml hawthorn (tincture strength 1:2) (for precautions see page 37)
- 20ml wild yam (tincture strength 1:2)
- 20ml vervain (tincture strength 1:2)
- 20ml St John's wort (tincture strength 1:2) (for precautions see page 85)

To make
- Mix ingredients together.
- Pour into a clean, dark glass bottle.
- Label with the contents and the date.
- Store at room temperature for up to a year.

Adult dose: 5ml diluted with some water, 2-3 times a day.

MIX FOR MENOPAUSAL SYMPTOMS (MAIN PROBLEM: MOOD SWINGS)

Ingredients
- 25ml rose (tincture strength 1:2)
- 25ml vervain (tincture strength 1:2)
- 25ml St John's wort (tincture strength 1:2) (for precautions see page 85)
- 25ml wild yam (tincture strength 1:2)

To make
- Mix ingredients together.
- Pour into a clean, dark glass bottle.
- Label with the contents and the date.
- Store at room temperature for up to a year.

Adult dose: 5ml, diluted with some water, 2-3 times a day.

Periods, heavy

Heavy periods can be due to fibroids or endometriosis, so it is worth having a proper check-up. If these problems are excluded, you can resort to the measures below. You may need to take Floradix or another iron supplement if your blood loss is very heavy.

Treatment options
- Take yarrow for a few months to achieve a sustained effect (for precautions see page 137). *Adults:* 2-4ml diluted with some water, 1-3 times a day, tincture strength 1:5; or 1-2 cups of yarrow tea a day.

- Take a large dose of shepherd's purse during the first 2 days of your period only (for precautions see page 140). *Adults:* 10ml diluted with some water 3-4 times a day, tincture strength 1:2; or 3-4 cups of tea a day.

Teenagers (10-16 years old): adjust the adult dose downwards, depending on the age of the teenager – see Chapter 6.

PERIODS, PAINFUL

Practitioner treatment is recommended for this condition.

Sorting out painful periods often requires a holistic approach, with a herbal prescription, improvements in one's diet and changes to one's lifestyle. There may be a specific hormonal imbalance that is best corrected by a medical herbalist. The measures below can be used during a period to ease the pain: commence taking the herbs on the day when the period pain starts. It is possible that you will feel sleepy with the dosages below; if so, try reducing the dose next time.

Treatment options

- Take valerian tincture. *Adults:* 5ml diluted with some water, 3-4 times a day for 2 days only, tincture strength 1:1.

- Take cramp bark tincture, by itself or as well as valerian. *Adults:* 2ml diluted with some water, 3-4 times a day for 2 days only, tincture strength 1:2.

- Drink strong chamomile tea (for precautions see page 114). *Adults:* 2-3 cups a day.

- Take the mix for reducing period pain – see box opposite.

Teenagers (10-16 years old): adjust the adult dose downwards, depending on the age of the teenager – see Chapter 6.

MIX FOR REDUCING PERIOD PAIN

Ingredients
- 20ml valerian (tincture strength 1:1)
- 30ml chamomile (tincture strength 1:5) (for precautions see page 114)
- 20ml cramp bark (tincture strength 1:2)
- 30ml yarrow (tincture strength 1:2) (for precautions see page 137)

To make
- Mix ingredients together.
- Pour into a clean, dark glass bottle.
- Label with the contents and the date.
- Store at room temperature for up to a year.

Adult dose: 5ml diluted with some water, 2-3 times a day for 3-6 months.

PMS (PREMENSTRUAL SYNDROME)

Practitioner treatment is recommended for this condition.

PMS is a combination of troublesome symptoms that some women experience before the onset of each period. These include: nervous tension, irritability, anger, low mood, sore breasts, bloated stomach, lack of concentration, and cravings for sugar and chocolate. There are many herbs that can help, but they need to be matched carefully to your individual symptoms.

Treatment options

- Take evening primrose oil in capsules. *Adults:* 3g daily from mid-cycle to the onset of your period.

- Take calming herbs such as valerian, chamomile (for precautions see page 114) or lemon balm, either singly or in combination (see Chapter 13, on the nervous system, for dosages). Take the herbs from mid-cycle to the onset of your period, and throughout the period itself.

- If you suffer from water retention (sore breasts, bloating) take dandelion leaf tea daily, starting 10 days before your period and stopping with the onset of your period. *Adults:* 2 cups a day.

Teenagers (11-16 years old): adjust the adult dose downwards, depending on the age of the teenager – see Chapter 6.

PROLAPSE

Uterine prolapse in its early stages and of recent origin can be improved with a simple herbal measure. There should normally be a rapid improvement within days or a couple of weeks, but to maintain the level of improvement reached you may have to continue the treatment for many months.

Treatment option

- Drink shepherd's purse tea on a daily basis (for precautions see page 140). *Adults only:* 2-3 cups a day.

THRUSH

Practitioner treatment is recommended for recurrent episodes.

Many women self-medicate for thrush with medicines available over the counter. Herbs can be very helpful, but if the problem recurs often, see a herbalist for a more individual approach. A helpful thing to do is to stop washing the genital area altogether for a few days – this allows the naturally present bacteria to multiply and compete with the thrush yeast.

Treatment options

- Take thyme tincture. *Adults:* 0.7-1.5ml, diluted with some water, 1-3 times a day, tincture strength 1:2.

- Take fresh garlic (for precautions see page 96). *Adults:* 1 clove crushed and mixed with honey, 1-2 times a day.

- Have a 'sitz bath' in a strong calendula infusion (for precautions see page 114). The term comes from the German 'to sit', and the idea is that you sit in a basin filled with the herbal infusion so that the relevant parts of the body come into contact with the herbs for several minutes. *Dose:* 2-3 times a day, for 5-10 minutes each time.

- Use the cream for thrush – see box overleaf.

- Take the mix for persisting thrush if it continues for longer than a week – see box overleaf.

Teenagers (11-16 years old): adjust the internal adult dose downwards, depending on the age of the teenager – see Chapter 6.

CREAM FOR THRUSH

Ingredients

- 20g calendula ointment (for precautions see page 114)
- 5 drops tea tree essential oil (for precautions see page 118)

To make

- Mix well.
- Transfer to a clean, dark glass jar, making sure that there are no air pockets left.
- Store for up to 12 months.

To use: apply 2-3 times a day, both inside and outside.

MIX FOR PERSISTING THRUSH

Ingredients

- 30ml thyme (tincture strength 1:2)
- 30ml calendula (tincture strength 1:2) (for precautions see page 114)
- 40ml white dead nettle (tincture strength 1:5)

To make

- Mix ingredients together.
- Pour into a clean, dark glass bottle.
- Label with the contents and the date.
- Store at room temperature for up to a year.

Adult dose: 5ml diluted with some water, 2-3 times a day.

WHEN AND WHY YOU SHOULD SEE A PROFESSIONAL MEDICAL HERBALIST

- Endometriosis: mild cases of this condition respond well to specific anti-inflammatory herbs.

- Severe menopausal symptoms: an individual combination of hormone-regulating herbs is required.

- Major problems with periods / severe PMS: many factors can be involved apart from hormonal imbalance, so careful assessment is needed.

- Polycystic ovary syndrome (PCOS): the treatment varies according to which particular health issues are present in a given woman with this condition.

- Kidney stones: if you have been diagnosed with kidney stones but don't need urgent treatment, it is worth trying specific herbs that have a reputation for dissolving small stones; herbs can be used to treat the colic caused by kidney stones but such herbs are available only to qualified practitioners.

- Low sex drive: often different herbs are used for males and females.

- Infertility / low sperm count: herbs can improve the ability to conceive but need to be prescribed individually for each case.

- Recurrent cystitis / interstitial cystitis / irritable bladder: these conditions may mimic each other; the treatment may take many months with many adjustments to the prescription.

- Pelvic inflammatory disease: strong antibacterial and anti-inflammatory herbs need to be used, so this is best done under supervision.

THE FOLLOWING SYMPTOMS WARRANT SEEING A HEALTH PROFESSIONAL WITHOUT DELAY

- Severe pain in your lower abdomen.

- High temperature (above 39°C/102°F) and dragging or stabbing pain in your lower abdomen (women: possible ectopic pregnancy).

- Women: any major change to your usual period pattern.

- Women: extreme bleeding during your period.

- Women: unusual discharge or bleeding, especially after the menopause.

- Men: unusual discharge from the urethra.

- Men: any enlargement of the testicles or a lump.

- Men: difficulty with and increased frequency of urinating.

- Pain around the loin area, especially if combined with cystitis, general malaise or running a high temperature (possible kidney infection).

- Colicky pain in the loins (possibly a kidney stone).

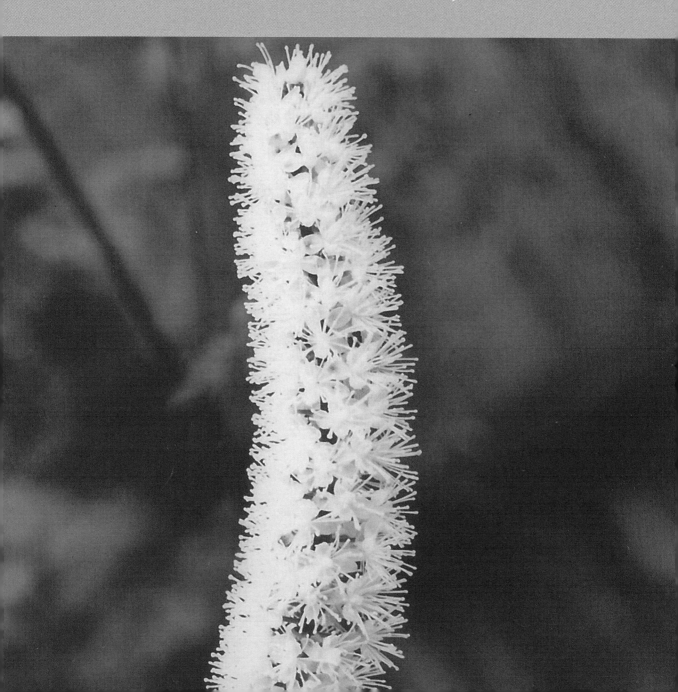

Part Three
Improving your vitality

Chapter 17

Maintain good energy levels

CHANGES IN ENERGY LEVELS

Many people complain about lack of energy. Our capacity to maintain high energy decreases naturally with age, and it is unrealistic to expect the same levels of energy from a 60-year-old as from a 20-year-old. You must make allowances for such a decrease as well as for the fact that some people are genetically more energetic than others. However, a drastic change in your normal energy levels does not occur without a reason.

COMMON CAUSES OF LOW ENERGY

- Overwork: this applies equally to a busy executive as to a mother looking after three young children.

- Prolonged stress: stress that continues for a long time can exhaust the adrenal glands, which help our bodies to respond to stress.

- Lack of sleep: this should be rather obvious, but many people expect to function well on an inadequate amount of sleep. A good night's sleep is essential for the body and the brain to recuperate after each day, especially a day that has been physically and mentally demanding.

- Faulty nutrition: food is the 'fuel' for your body in a literal sense – our energy comes from oxidising (i.e. 'burning') glucose, which comes from the food we eat. However, to produce the molecules that are energy carriers, body cells need many vitamins and minerals. If these are lacking, which is often the case in a modern, highly processed diet, the body simply cannot maintain an adequate production of energy. One of the most common nutritional problems leading to lack of energy is drinking too much coffee.

- Depression: poor energy, perhaps better described as lethargy, is one of the symptoms of depression.

- Disease: many diseases result in low energy; even a bad cold can leave you exhausted for weeks. It is always worth checking whether your thyroid is working properly, as it is the thyroid that determines your basic metabolic rate, which in turn influences your level of energy.

- Lack of exercise: exercise stimulates the circulation in your body and the supply of oxygen and nutrients to your brain. If you don't move much, such vital supplies will be sluggish and you will feel sluggish too.

IDENTIFY THE CAUSE AND TREAT IT

This is not an exhaustive list – there can be many more reasons or combinations of factors, and you need to identify precisely what the underlying problem is in your case. Some health problems causing low energy, such as depression, insomnia or post-viral fatigue, are discussed in other chapters, so please refer to these as necessary and treat the conditions with the suggested herbs. Attending to the possible causes should be your first line of approach, before reaching straight away for energising herbs. Some ailments, such as low thyroid function, will necessitate seeing a health professional and taking appropriate medication, whether herbal or conventional.

HERBS AND LIFESTYLE ADJUSTMENTS

The herbs discussed below are energy boosters, and are suitable for people who need an extra 'oomph' for a short period of time – say a few days to a few months.

However, there is no point in taking herbs to improve your energy if you do not make essential lifestyle adjustments – the herbs can prop you up for a while, but unless you deal with the cause of your tiredness the problem will come back.

I cannot stress enough that herbs are not a substitute for a healthy lifestyle, sensible working hours and a good diet. Energy-boosting herbs will work up to a point, but if you continually push your body to the point of exhaustion and give it no chance to recover, even the best herbs will stop working.

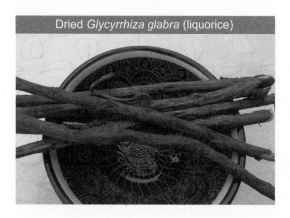
Dried *Glycyrrhiza glabra* (liquorice)

THE HERBS TO CHOOSE FROM

SIBERIAN GINSENG

Warning: Do not take during the acute phase of an infection.

Uses
Siberian ginseng belongs to the group of herbs called adaptogens. Such herbs help the body to adapt to stress, whether physical or mental. They do so by improving the functioning of all the body's systems, which makes the whole organism more resilient to stress. The results are perceived as better energy, better functioning, better concentration, better memory, better endurance and better immune responses. This enhancement of physical and mental abilities leads to greater levels of efficiency in performing a particular task, which should leave you more time for proper rest. In fact, sleep becomes deeper and more refreshing as well. Overall, not only do you start feeling more energetic but you can also do more in a shorter time.

Siberian ginseng is a true all-round tonic, suitable for adults and children, which can be taken for many months if necessary.

Combinations
It combines well with liquorice, relaxing or antidepressant herbs (e.g. St John's wort, vervain, valerian, lemon balm) and herbs modulating the immune system (e.g. echinacea). Refer to the appropriate chapters for information on these herbs.

How to take
As a tincture.

Dosage
Adults: 1-4ml diluted with some water, 1-2 times a day, tincture strength 1:2.
Children (8-16 years old): adjust the adult dose downwards, depending on the age of the child – see Chapter 6.

ASHWAGANDA

Uses
Ashwaganda, an Ayurvedic herb which can be cultivated in the UK, is also an adaptogen. Its range of actions is similar to that of Siberian ginseng, but it also includes anti-inflammatory and mild sedative properties. This herb would make a better choice for somebody whose low energy arises from illness, either current or recent (e.g. depression, cancer, influenza, chronic fatigue syndrome or anaemia). It also helps to rebuild muscle strength after a period of physical inactivity. You can use this herb on its own to improve your energy or in a mix that will address other aspects of your health. Ashwaganda can be taken for long periods of time.

How to take
As a tincture.

Dosage
Adults: 1.5-3.5ml diluted with some water, 1-2 times a day, tincture strength 1:1.
Children (8-16 years old): adjust the adult dose downwards, depending on the age of the child – see Chapter 6.

KOREAN GINSENG

Warning: Do not use if suffering from an acute disease or high blood pressure.
Not suitable for children.
Caution: best avoided if taking warfarin, antidepressants, coffee or other stimulants.

Uses
This tonic herb of Chinese origin should be used wisely, as it can over-stimulate the body. Traditionally it was given mainly to men over 40 as an energy and vitality booster. In my experience, Korean ginseng is more suitable for mature people than for those who are younger, and should be taken for only short periods of time, from a few days to a month. I recommend it for loss of energy related to ageing, but you can use it as a stronger-acting substitute for Siberian ginseng or ashwaganda for short periods of time.

If you feel lightheaded or hyperactive and develop a fast heart rate, you must reduce the dose.

How to take
As tablets or tincture.

Dosage
Adults: 300-500mg a day (tablet form); or 0.5-2.5ml diluted with some water, 2 times a day, tincture strength 1:2.

LIQUORICE

Caution needed when pregnant or if elderly. Do not take if you have high blood pressure, low potassium, heart or kidney or liver problems, or water retention.

Uses

Liquorice is an adrenal tonic, and as such it is an apt choice for treating adrenal exhaustion owing to continuous stress. It provides supportive treatment when lack of energy results from unrelenting stressful pressures, and is exceptionally useful if the stress has had a negative effect on one's digestion. I recommend it for people who work exceptionally long hours and are under constant pressure to deliver results. It is also suited for low-energy situations resulting from disease (e.g. chronic fatigue syndrome).

Combinations

I strongly recommend combining liquorice with a relaxing herb of your choice. It also mixes well with Siberian ginseng or ashwaganda.

How to take

As a tincture.

Dosage

Adults: 0.4-1.6ml diluted with some water, 1-3 times a day, tincture strength 1:1.
Children (3-16 years old): adjust the adult dose downwards, depending on the age of the child – see Chapter 6.

STRATEGY FOR IMPROVING ENERGY LEVELS

- Treat the underlying health problem that is causing low energy.

- Add a herb or herbs that improve energy.

- Use restorative herbs that gradually restore health to a malfunctioning system or organ, e.g. oats for the nervous system, echinacea for the immune system, etc.

The example mix in the box shows one of the possible combinations. Remember that this formula may not suit your individual situation.

EXAMPLE MIX FOR IMPROVING ENERGY LEVELS

Ingredients
- 20ml St John's wort (tincture strength 1:2) (for precautions see page 85)
- 20ml Siberian ginseng (tincture strength 1:2) (for precautions see page 152)
- 20ml ashwaganda (tincture strength 1:1)
- 20ml oats (tincture strength 1:2)
- 20ml vervain (tincture strength 1:2)

To make
- Mix ingredients together.
- Pour into a clean, dark glass bottle.
- Label with the contents and the date.
- Store at room temperature for up to a year.

Adult dose: 5ml, diluted with some water, 2-3 times a day.
Children (8-16 years old): adjust the adult dose downwards, depending on the age of the child – see Chapter 6.

Chapter 18
Increase your mental and physical stamina

There is an overlap in herbal use for the improvement of general energy levels and the improvement of levels of stamina and endurance. I suggest that you read Chapter 17 to see if any of the described herbs and herbal strategies are applicable to your individual circumstances.

WHEN TO USE HERBS

In this chapter I focus on a particular aspect of human functioning – that of mental and physical stamina. There are plenty of situations in modern life that require extra performance: for example, we have exams, deadlines at work, sick children who won't sleep, a sports event, etc. They all tap into our natural reserves of energy, but these reserves can be gently enhanced with the help of specific herbs. In effect, you will be able to study more intensively and for a longer period of time, concentrate on your task better and perform better in your chosen sport.

MATCHING HERBS TO YOUR SITUATION

The underlying principle of herbal use for these purposes is to improve the general functioning of the body with the help of tonic herbs and to improve the functioning of specific body systems involved in a particular activity that requires extra effort. Let me give you a couple of examples: if you have a very difficult exam and you need to study excep-

tionally hard, you will want to combine energy boosters with herbs that improve circulation to the brain and improve the quality of sleep. If you are going to trek for many days at a high altitude, you will want a general tonic, plus warming herbs that aid general circulation, plus herbs that aid the recovery of joints and muscles overnight.

SHORT-TERM VERSUS LONG-TERM USE

It is important to understand the difference between a short, intense boost and prolonged, sustained use of herbs. Siberian ginseng and ashwaganda can be used long-term, for many months, while Korean ginseng should be a short-term measure – a few days to up to a month. For short-term action, use maximum doses of these herbs; for long-term go for the medium-to-low end of the dose. An intense boost should be used only in exceptional circumstances.

THE HERBS TO CHOOSE FROM

- Siberian ginseng, or ashwaganda, or Korean ginseng (see pages 152 and 153): all three herbs are improvers of mental and physical performance and stamina.

- Liquorice (see page 154), if you have been under a lot of stress for a while.

- Ginkgo and hawthorn (see pages 36 and 37): examples of circulatory improvers.

- Arnica, comfrey and rosemary (see pages 68, 69 and 71): examples of aids in recovery from physical strain.

HERBAL STRATEGY TO IMPROVE PERFORMANCE AND STAMINA

- Choose one or two suitable adaptogen herbs (see Chapter 17).

- Add liquorice (see page 154) if you already feel low on energy.

- Add herbs that improve circulation (see Chapter 10).

EXAMPLE MIX FOR IMPROVING PHYSICAL STAMINA

Ingredients
- 30ml Korean ginseng (tincture strength 1:2) (for precautions see page 153)
- 20ml ginger (tincture strength 1:2) (for precautions see page 52)
- 30ml ashwaganda (tincture strength 1:1)
- 20ml ginkgo (tincture strength 1:2) (for precautions see page 36)

To make
- Mix ingredients together.
- Pour into a clean, dark glass bottle.
- Label with the contents and the date.
- Store at room temperature for up to a year.

Adults only: 5ml, diluted with some water, 2 times a day.

- Add herbs that improve physical recovery from strenuous exercise (see Chapter 12).

The example mixes in the boxes show some of the possible combinations, but remember that these formulae may not suit your individual situation.

EXAMPLE MIX FOR IMPROVING MENTAL PERFORMANCE

Ingredients
- 20ml ginkgo (tincture strength 1:2) (for precautions see page 36)
- 30ml Siberian ginseng (tincture strength 1:2) (for precautions see page 152)
- 30ml ashwaganda (tincture strength 1:1)
- 20ml liquorice (tincture strength 1:1) (for precautions see page 154)

To make
- Mix ingredients together.
- Pour into a clean, dark glass bottle.
- Label with the contents and the date.
- Store at room temperature for up to a year.

Adults only: 5ml diluted with some water, 2-3 times a day.

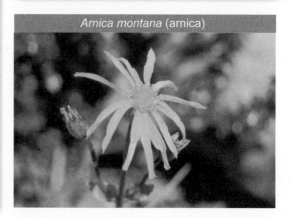
Arnica montana (arnica)

EXAMPLE CREAM TO AID MUSCLE AND JOINT RECOVERY AFTER STRENUOUS EXERCISE

Ingredients
- 20g comfrey cream
- 10g arnica cream
- 10ml of wild yam tincture
- 10 drops rosemary essential oil (for precautions see page 71)
- 10 drops wintergreen essential oil (for precautions see page 74)
- 5 drops lavender essential oil (for precautions see page 72)

To make
- Mix well.
- Transfer to a clean, dark glass jar, making sure that there are no air pockets left.
- Store for up to 12 months.

Adults and children over 3 years old: apply to the aching muscles or joints 1-2 times a day or straight after exercise.

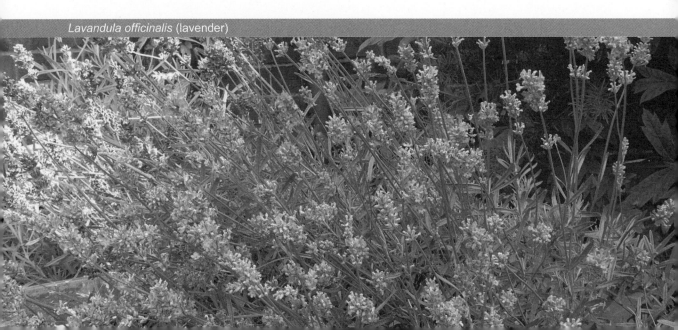

Lavandula officinalis (lavender)

Chapter 19

Revive your libido

CAUSES OF LOW LIBIDO

Low sex drive can result from many factors, for example, age, tiredness, illness or relationship problems. As always, you need to look at the possible reasons and address those before resorting to aphrodisiac herbs. It is natural to lose interest in sex as we age, and as long as both partners are happy with this decline there should be no problem.

Many illnesses and associated conventional treatments can diminish the libido, so make sure you are well informed about your symptoms and the side effects of your medication. Herbs are unlikely to override the effects of such medication, so you may want to look for alternatives from your doctor (or consider herbal treatment for your original ailment). The most common condition that has a negative effect on sex drive is depression. The second most common is overwork and lack of sleep!

WHAT HERBS CAN DO

Where herbs can help is to put you in a generally happy frame of mind, give you more energy, relax you, improve the blood supply to your vital organs and gently stimulate interest in sex.

LENGTH OF TREATMENT

The treatment should be relatively short-term – a month or two. If you don't see any difference in your libido after that time, consider seeing a herbalist, who may be able to sort out the underlying causes, especially if they are related to hormonal imbalances.

THE HERBS TO CHOOSE FROM

- Siberian ginseng, ashwaganda (see pages 152 and 153): general energy improvers.

- Korean ginseng (see page 153): improves the libido in older people.

- Damiana (see page 139): a gentle mood and libido improver for younger people.

- Vervain, St John's wort (see pages 55 and 85): antidepressants and mood improvers.

- Hawthorn, ginkgo, ginger (see pages 36, 37 and 52): circulatory herbs.

- Valerian, lemon balm, passionflower (see pages 81, 53 and 85): sleep-improving herbs.

- Essential oils with stimulating qualities: nutmeg, labdanum, sandalwood, rose, cinnamon leaf, myrrh, cedar (for precautions see pages 23 and 26).

HERBAL STRATEGY TO IMPROVE LIBIDO

- Combine one of the energy improvers with one of the libido improvers as a basic treatment.

- Add a relaxant or a mood improver if anxiety or low mood are an issue.

- Add a circulatory herb if you don't get much exercise or have problems with blood circulation.

- Improve your sleep with a dedicated sleep mix (see page 90).

- Invest in one or two good-quality essential oils that can put you and your partner in the right mood; use them in a relaxing bath or add to a massage oil. For precautions see pages 23 and 26.

The example mix in the box shows one of the possible combinations, but remember that this formula may not suit your individual situation.

EXAMPLE MIX FOR IMPROVING LIBIDO

Ingredients

- 20ml damiana (tincture strength 1:2) (for precautions see page 139)
- 20ml Korean ginseng (tincture strength 1:2) (for precautions see page 153)
- 20ml ashwaganda (tincture strength 1:1)
- 20ml hawthorn (tincture strength 1:2) (for precautions see page 37)
- 20ml lemon balm (tincture strength 1:2)

To make

- Mix ingredients together.
- Pour into a clean, dark glass bottle.
- Label with the contents and the date.
- Store at room temperature for up to a year.

Adults only: 5ml diluted with some water, 2-3 times a day.

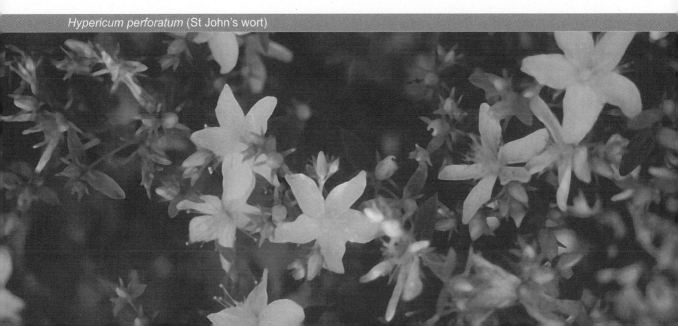

Hypericum perforatum (St John's wort)

Chapter 20
Feel motivated and happy

CAUSES OF UNHAPPINESS

You don't need to be depressed in order to act to improve your mood and motivation: many herbs are gentle mood enhancers suitable for people whose enthusiasm for life is not as strong as it used to be. I strongly believe that the natural state of mind is contentment. Of course there are objective reasons why we become unhappy – for example illness, job or relationship stress, or money worries – but there are also many other reasons, often unappreciated by the unhappy individual, such as lack of exercise, the way one lives and eats, lack of contact with nature, no hobbies or interests, and fixed attitudes as to what constitutes happiness.

Sometimes, however, we become dissatisfied with life for no apparent reason. Our zest for life diminishes and we don't feel like doing anything.

LONG-TERM VERSUS SHORT-TERM TREATMENT

If you are in the former category you will need to look carefully at your life and change those things that influence your mood negatively. You can resort to the herbs described below while trying to sort things out. You may need to use these herbs for a longer period of time (two to six months).

If you are in the latter category, a short course of treatment (a few days to a couple of weeks) with some of the herbs described below should restore your former enthusiasm

for life. Once you feel happier, you won't need the herbs any more. The herbs should put you in the right frame of mind, and once that is achieved it should be a self-perpetuating state.

THE HERBS TO CHOOSE FROM

- Ashwaganda (see page 153): this herb puts the mind in a positive frame and improves motivation.

- Rose (see page 85), damiana (see page 139), vervain (see page 55): these herbs are gentle mood improvers.

- Oats (see page 84): a restorative herb for the nervous system.

- Ginkgo (see page 36), ginger (see page 52), hawthorn (see page 37): circulation improvers.

HERBAL STRATEGY TO IMPROVE YOUR FEELING OF WELL-BEING

- Take ashwaganda as a choice adaptogen herb.

- Add one or two mood improvers.

- Add oats if the problem has been a long-standing one.

- Add a circulatory herb (see Chapter 10) if you don't do much exercise – but try to introduce some exercise into your lifestyle.

The example mix in the box shows one of the possible combinations, but remember that this formula may not suit your individual situation.

EXAMPLE MIX FOR IMPROVING A SENSE OF WELL-BEING

Ingredients

- 20ml ginkgo (tincture strength 2:1) (for precautions see page 36)
- 20ml ashwaganda (tincture strength 1:1)
- 20ml oats (tincture strength 1:2)
- 20ml vervain (tincture strength 1:2)
- 20ml damiana (tincture strength 1:2) (for precautions see page 139)

To make

- Mix ingredients together.
- Pour into a clean, dark glass bottle.
- Label with the contents and the date.
- Store at room temperature for up to a year.

Adults only: 5ml diluted with some water, 2-3 times a day.

Note: this mix is suitable for both short- and long-term use.

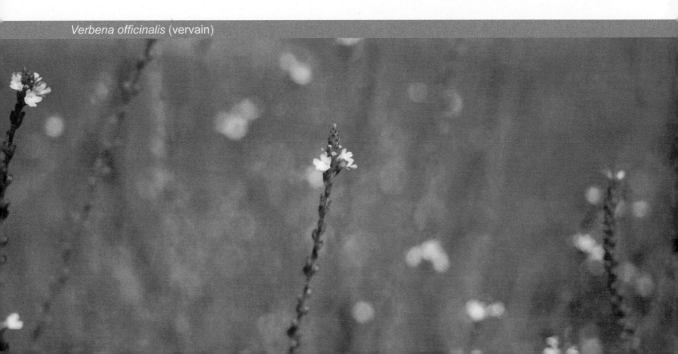

Verbena officinalis (vervain)

Chapter 21
Defy the ageing process

We all want to live long and enjoy good health. Herbs can greatly enhance your chances of slowing down or preventing many of the degenerative conditions so common in older people: heart disease, stroke, cancer, dementia and inflammatory diseases (respiratory or arthritic).

Of course, taking care of your body and mind in terms of good diet, regular exercise, keeping your weight down, avoiding stress and continuing mental activity are all vital. However, adding a few super-herbs (some of them being super-foods) to your health routine will substantially reduce the odds of a serious disease.

The following choice of herbs is for your own consideration, to be introduced on a daily basis if possible. Each of these herbs has merits in its own right and some of them may be more desirable than others in your particular situation; for instance, if there is a history of heart disease in your family you may consider taking garlic daily from the age of 30 onwards.

THE HERBS AND FOODS TO CHOOSE FROM

BLUEBERRIES

Anti-ageing benefits
Owing to their antioxidants, blueberries

prevent degenerative changes in the brain and circulatory system. Regular consumption of blueberries can bring about improvement in both night and day vision and avert the degeneration of the retina.

Dosage
Adults: 50-100g of berries a day or dry powder equivalent. For more information see page 36.

GINKGO

For precautions see page 36.

Anti-ageing benefits
Ginkgo protects the nerve cells from oxidative damage, improves the supply of oxygen to the brain, has anti-inflammatory and anti-allergic properties, enhances concentration and memory in healthy elderly people, and may play a role in preventing the onset of dementia.

Dosage
Adults: 2ml a day diluted with some water, tincture strength 2:1.

KOREAN GINSENG

For precautions see page 153.

Anti-ageing benefits
Korean ginseng has a protective effect against cancer, improves survival rates once the

cancer is in remission and increases general levels of vitality in mature people.

Dosage
Adults: 2ml a day, diluted with some water, tincture strength 1:2; you need to take it frequently, though not daily, or on a month on/month off basis. Take the tablets according to the manufacturer's instructions.

GARLIC

For precautions see page 52.

Anti-ageing benefits
Garlic lessens the risk of cardiovascular disease in relation to a wide range of factors, including reducing the formation of fatty plaques in the arteries, preserving arterial-wall elasticity, lowering blood pressure and cholesterol, and reducing the tendency for blood clot formation and the frequency of viral infections. Fresh crushed garlic can be eaten in salads, or mixed with houmous or honey.

Dosage
Adults: about 5g of fresh garlic a day; or an enteric-coated tablet containing 5.7mg of alliin a day.

ECHINACEA

For precautions see page 137.

Anti-ageing benefits
Echinacea reduces the number of viral and bacterial infections, which play a role in many degenerative illnesses.

Dosage
Adults: 1-2ml diluted with some water, 2-3 times a day, tincture strength 1:5.

HAWTHORN

For precautions see page 37.

Anti-ageing benefits
Hawthorn improves the functioning of the circulatory system, especially the circulation to the heart and brain, and lowers blood pressure.

Dosage
Adults: 1-2ml diluted with some water, 1-3 times a day, tincture strength 1:5.

GREEN TEA

Anti-ageing benefits
Regular consumption of green tea is associated with lower incidence of various cancers, the enhanced survival of cancer patients, decreased risk of cardiovascular disease and prevention of memory decline in elderly people.

Dosage
Adults: 3-5 cups a day; do not add milk. Alternatively, take as capsules of green tea extract according to the manufacturer's instructions.

OTHER ANTI-AGEING FOODS AND PLANTS

Other foods that can help defy the ageing process include: red grape juice, red wine, grape seed extract, turmeric, olive oil, hemp seed oil, linseed oil.

Chapter 22
Make a full recovery from a serious illness

A serious illness can take a toll on the body, and it often takes weeks or months to achieve a full recovery. A suitable choice of herbs can greatly enhance the recovery process, but you must match such herbs carefully to your circumstances. Recovering from illness also means taking things easy, eating nutritious food and resting a lot. The temptation may be to start charging around as soon as you feel better after taking some herbs. Do resist this to begin with, and allow plenty of rest for a few days or even weeks if your disease has been long-lasting.

The herbs given below are the most commonly used for convalescence from a variety of problems. You may look up other herbs that are recommended in connection with particular diseases and add those to your choice: for instance, after surgery you may want to use skin healers or arnica. Recovering from cancer is a special category and I recommend seeing a herbalist for that.

Post-viral fatigue or chronic fatigue syndrome (often called ME) are effectively symptoms of an incomplete recovery from an illness. If your fatigue has been relatively short-term (3-6 months), follow the general strategy below for 2-3 months. If you have been suffering for more than 6 months, I suggest seeing a herbalist because you will need a more complex, individualised treatment.

THE HERBS TO CHOOSE FROM

- Elderflower, calendula, propolis, garlic (see pages 95, 114, 99 and 52): antiviral herbs.

- Thyme, propolis, barberry, garlic (see pages 100, 99, 51 and 52): antibacterial herbs.

- Echinacea (see page 98): an immune modulator.

- Ashwaganda (see page 153): use this herb if there has been some body wasting as a result of disease and your general levels of vitality are low.

- Liquorice (see page 53): the herb for adrenal exhaustion.

- Vervain, St John's wort, rose, oats (see pages 55, 85 and 84): antidepressants and restoratives to the nervous system.

- Siberian ginseng (see page 152): an improver of vitality and energy.

HERBAL STRATEGY TO AID RECOVERY FROM ILLNESS

- If you are suffering from an infectious illness, choose one or two antiviral/ antibacterial herbs and start taking these at the maximum recommended dose for 7-10 days.

- If you have had an infectious illness it is still worth taking one or two antiviral/antibacterial herbs at the medium recommended dose (7-10 days) to eradicate the bug.

- Prop up your immune system with echinacea if you are over the acute phase of your illness.

- Take ashwaganda if you have lost too much weight due to illness.

- Take ashwaganda and/or Siberian ginseng if your energy levels are low (however, do not take these if you are still very ill).

- Take liquorice if your disease has been long-lasting and has left you mentally and physically exhausted.

- Take one or two herbs that improve mood if your illness has left you feeling low, lethargic or depressed.

EXAMPLE MIX FOR IMPROVING THE RECOVERY FROM INFECTIOUS ILLNESS

Ingredients

- 20ml St John's wort (tincture strength 1:2) (for precautions see page 85)
- 20ml Siberian ginseng (tincture strength 1:2) (for precautions see page 152)
- 20ml ashwaganda (tincture strength 1:1)
- 20ml propolis (tincture strength 1:2) (for precautions see page 99)
- 20ml vervain (tincture strength 1:2)

To make

- Mix ingredients together.
- Pour into a clean, dark glass bottle.
- Label with the contents and the date.
- Store at room temperature for up to a year.

Adults: 5ml diluted with some water, 2-3 times a day.

Children (8-16 years old): adjust the adult dose downwards, depending on the age of the child – see Chapter 6.

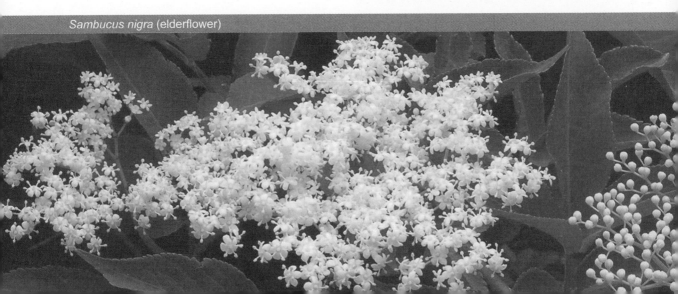

Sambucus nigra (elderflower)

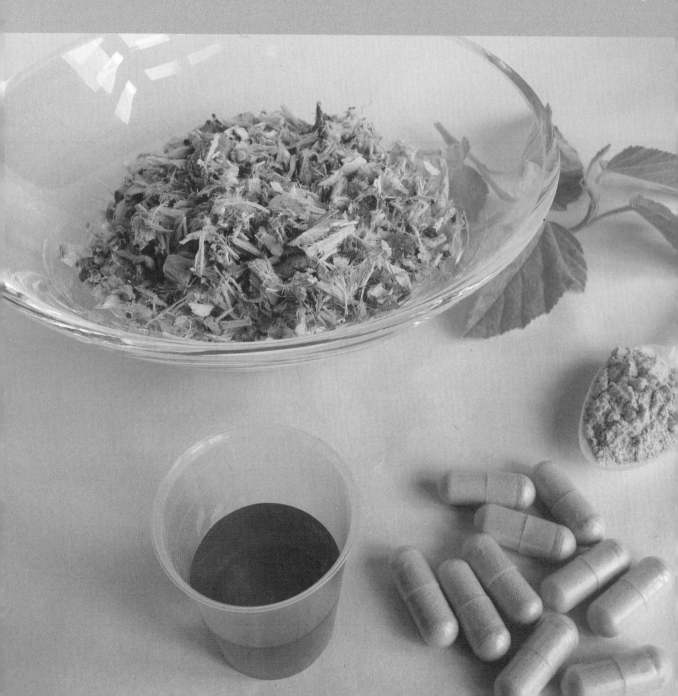

Part Four
Creating your own home apothecary

Chapter 23
Buying from reputable sources

BUYING VERSUS GROWING

If you want to stock herbs for regular use you have two options: you can either grow your own or buy from herbal suppliers.

I would like to encourage you to grow your own, but I recognise that most people are too busy to dry their own herbs or to make their own tinctures. I think that for the majority of people a compromise solution will work best: you may want to grow a few herbs that are easy to cultivate and versatile in use, to maybe make a herbal syrup or ointment, but otherwise you may prefer to buy ready-made herbal products.

Whichever you choose, there are some important issues associated with both growing and buying. The pros and cons of buying are discussed in this chapter, while the advantages of growing your own and suggestions for the choice of herbs to grow are given in Chapter 24.

ADVANTAGES OF BUYING READY-MADE PRODUCTS

The main advantages of buying from herbal suppliers are: ready-made tinctures are often superior in quality to home-made versions (some manufactures will check the actual biochemical composition of each batch to ensure consistent quality), you can buy larger quantities if necessary, you can buy herbs in tablet form that cannot be made at home, and you have access to a wide variety of herbs, some of which cannot be grown in the British climate.

PROBLEMS ASSOCIATED WITH READY-MADE PRODUCTS

There are, however, some issues associated with ready-made herbal products. Unscrupulous traders will sell adulterated products, where one plant species has been substituted for another. Such adulteration can be seriously harmful, if potentially toxic plants are used as substitutes. Some herbal preparations on the market are of poor quality and will have little therapeutic value, while others are artificially 'strengthened' with a particular constituent and the safety of such products is unknown.

Therefore when you decide to buy ready-processed herbs, consider the points below in order to be safe and not waste your money.

BUY FROM REPUTABLE SUPPLIERS ONLY

This is paramount. You should buy only from suppliers that can guarantee the quality of their products. Please refer to the Resources section for the list of retailers and suppliers to choose from. As a rule of thumb, obtain your herbs from well-known companies: the European and Australian companies making herbal products have the best reputation. Do not buy online unless the site is run by a genuine herbalist who is a member of a recognised herbal association (see page 196). Unfortunately, not all health food shops can be relied on to offer consistent high quality across the herbal product range.

BUY DIRECTLY FROM HERBAL APOTHECARIES

Many bona fide medical herbalists run their own apothecaries, and these are the best sources from which to buy your herbs as you will be guaranteed good quality, plus you will receive advice on the appropriate dosage. To find such apothecaries, contact the organisations listed on page 196.

BUY NATIVE HERBS OR CULTIVATED LOCALLY

Remember that herbs that are prone to adulteration are the imported, rare and exotic ones. Be aware that there is hardly any quality control of Chinese and Ayurvedic preparations at the moment, and there are frequently cases of herb adulteration in China and India. Buying native herbs or those that are non-native but cultivated in the UK reduces the risk of buying the wrong, and possibly harmful, species.

PRICE AND QUALITY

Price is often a reflection of quality – beware of exceptionally cheap products. However, an exorbitant price is not a guarantee of extra quality; most likely it means that the herb you are buying is rare and endangered. For ordinary herbs, you should currently expect to pay about £7-9 for 100ml of tincture and about half that for 100g of dry herbs, although that may depend on the actual species.

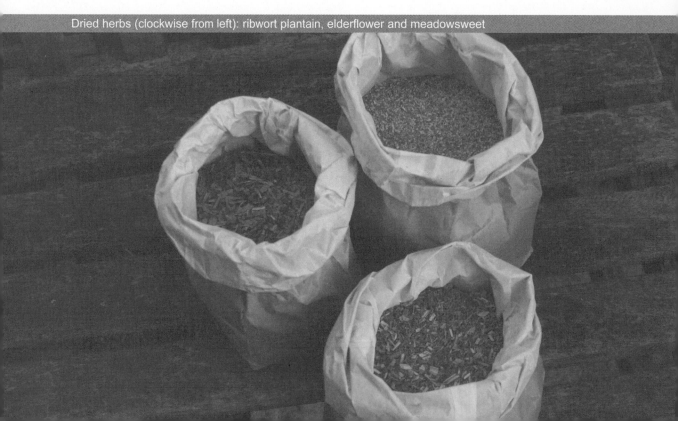
Dried herbs (clockwise from left): ribwort plantain, elderflower and meadowsweet

Chapter 24
Growing your own herbs

Before you start growing your own herbs you should ask yourself which herbs you will really use and how much of them you will need. Do you want to have just a few fragrant leaves to pick for a summer tea or do you want to make your own tinctures and creams?

HOW MUCH AND WHICH HERBS TO GROW

In general I recommend cultivating about 8-11 herbs that are exceptionally versatile, are available fresh for most of the year or are easy to dry. These herbs are included in List 1 in this chapter. For an average family you will not need many plants of each category: perhaps one lemon balm plant, one elderflower bush, 4-5 meadowsweet plants and a total of one square metre sown with chamomile or calendula (marigold). Many herbs, e.g. lemon balm, peppermint and calendula, can be repeatedly harvested through the season, which will encourage new growth. It is difficult to recommend a particular amount to grow, as needs will differ from family to family. As a general principle, plants that are evergreen and can be harvested all year round can be planted in small numbers, while plants that need to be dried or processed into tinctures will be required in bigger amounts.

EASY TO GROW

Herbs are the easiest plants to grow. They are generally undemanding in terms of soil and are robust and resistant to pests. Most are perennials, one or two are biennials and there are a few reliably self-seeding annuals. It is a joy to have your own lemon balm or peppermint for a refreshing and relaxing summer tea, and it is a pleasure to see the cheerful flowers of calendula open and close daily. Hawthorn and elderflower make much more graceful hedges than does leylandii, and they will be bustling with wildlife.

ORGANIC OR BIODYNAMIC

Herbs should be grown organically, which means no spraying of any kind. They don't need any fertiliser, natural or not – they prefer poor soil. Make sure the soil has not been contaminated with anything beforehand. If you intend to harvest the herbs from your garden for your own use it is worth reading up on biodynamic gardening and following the advice given – herbs grown and harvested along biodynamic lines have higher levels of active constituents.

ATTRACTING WILDLIFE

Flowering herbs provide a rich source of nectar for bees and butterflies, and some flower late into the season when not much insect food is around. Bushes that are used medicinally have both attractive flowers and valuable berries for the birds. You will be growing plants that happen to have medicinal value, while at the same time creating a wildflower garden.

WAYS TO GROW HERBS

You can grow your herbs in an organised, flowerbed fashion. You can grow them in pots. You can dot them around your garden or allotment between other plants and vegetables. In fact, they will be happiest when squeezed among other plants and made to struggle a bit – that's how they have to survive naturally. You can grow most herbs recommended in this book, apart from one or two which require a hot climate. And you do not need to grow them just to use them – many medicinal plants can be grown for their beauty or for their attractiveness to wildlife.

My preferred way of growing herbs is to have them mixed with other plants, either in the borders or in the vegetable plot. I grow marigold and chamomile between rows of carrots and radishes, I let the peppermint invade the raspberry bed and I plant black cohosh for its beautiful scented flowers to brighten late autumn. I have never planted St John's wort, elderflower, evening primrose, hawthorn, dandelion, nettles or ribwort plantain in my garden – they all came of their own accord, with the help of wind and birds, and I let them be, occasionally shifting a particular plant to a different place.

CULINARY HERBS

Of course there is also an overlap between culinary and medicinal herbs. You may grow certain herbs primarily for cooking and resort to their medicinal use only occasionally. Herbs in this category include garlic, dill, fennel, sage, thyme, peppermint, lavender and rosemary.

GROWING FROM SEEDS AND BUYING FROM NURSERIES

It is easy to grow herbs from seed, which you should get from specialist seed producers. You can also get mature plants from specialist nurseries. The varieties of herbs found in ordinary garden centres are often modified garden cultivars, which are also often incorrectly labelled. Remember to check the Latin name on the seed packet or plant label. Once you start growing annual herbs, collect the seeds or let the plants seed naturally. Some herbs (e.g. lemon balm, peppermint) need dividing or thinning out every few years, but most will live happily undisturbed in the same place without watering or fertilising. However, if cultivated in pots, herbs will need watering and an occasional soil boost (comfrey liquid manure being the best). Refer to the Resources section for the names of specialist nurseries.

RECOMMENDED SELECTION

Below I recommend a number of herbs to grow in your garden that can be easily harvested fresh and easily preserved. Another list gives you a choice of pretty herbs that flower nicely and can be incorporated into a perennial border. Then there is a list of herbs that have to be dug out to harvest the roots – they may need a dedicated place in your garden. Finally, I list those herbs that will appear uninvited in your lawn or a neglected corner of your garden, and which you should cherish and leave alone – once you know that they are valuable medicine that you can use if needed, you will no longer perceive them as useless weeds!

Refer to the Latin names list in Appendix 1 for harvesting times.

LIST 1: MUST-HAVES

These herbs are nice to have fresh, easy to harvest and dry, and versatile in use.

- Calendula
- Chamomile
- Elderflower
- Lavender
- Lemon balm
- Meadowsweet
- Peppermint
- Rose
- Rosemary
- Sage
- Thyme

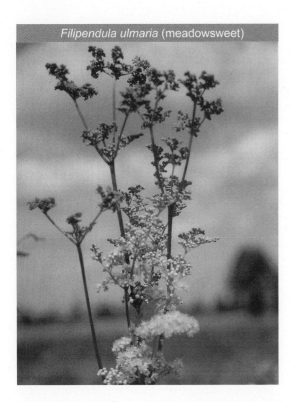

Filipendula ulmaria (meadowsweet)

LIST 2: PRETTY PLANTS / FLOWERS

The herbs in this list can be incorporated into the borders or hedging.

- Barberry
- Black cohosh
- Calendula
- Comfrey
- Cramp bark bush
- Echinacea
- Elecampane
- Evening primrose
- Eyebright
- Fennel
- Flax (linseed)
- Ginkgo tree
- Hawthorn
- Hops
- Lime tree
- Marshmallow
- Milk thistle
- Mountain grape
- St John's wort
- Valerian
- Wintergreen
- Witch hazel

LIST 3: ROOT HERBS

These herbs may need a dedicated place in your garden.

- Dandelion
- Echinacea
- Elecampane
- Valerian
- Yellow dock

LIST 4: WEEDS OR MEDICINE?

The herbs below happen to be common garden weeds, which will appear uninvited in your garden – perhaps let them grow in less conspicuous places with the view of occasional medicinal use.

- Dandelion
- Ground ivy
- Nettles
- Oats
- Red clover
- Ribwort plantain
- Shepherd's purse
- Vervain
- White deadnettle
- Yarrow

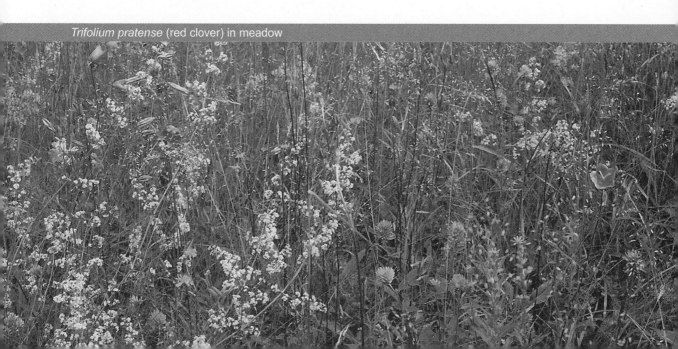

Trifolium pratense (red clover) in meadow

Chapter 25
Drying herbs

Drying herbs is the simplest way to preserve them. There are different ways to dry different parts of the plant, but the underlying process is the same: you expose cut herbs to heat so that the natural water content can evaporate. Because the British climate is so humid, I recommend that you use only the oven method, otherwise you are likely to end up with a half-mouldy product. Herbs need to be dried quickly, in reasonably high temperature and away from sunlight. Hanging bunches of herbs in the kitchen or attic looks picturesque but is not a good way to dry them – not enough air circulates around the herbs and they take too long to dry, which creates an opportunity for fungi to grow on the leaves.

If you intend to dry herbs you must collect the aerial parts (leaves, flowers, etc.) on a dry, sunny day; it's even better if you can do so after a few successive days without rain. It is not so important to collect the roots on a dry day, however, as you will still need to wash them. The aerial parts of herbs you gather must look healthy, without any visible disease or insect damage, and free from dirt so that you don't need to wash them.

Different herbs have different optimum times for harvesting, and following biodynamic principles of sowing and harvesting will yield better-quality herbs. See the list of common herbs in Appendix 1 for harvesting times.

PREPARE THE APPROPRIATE PART

- Parts of the plant above ground should be left for a while after harvesting to give any small insects a chance to crawl away. Then chop the leaves and stems roughly with a sharp knife or herb rocking knife.

- Flowers need to be cut off the stems. In the case of calendula and rose, detach the petals. Flowers that produce large umbels, such as elderflower, should be dried with the stems but then shaken off. Small flowers such as chamomile should be dried whole with a bit of stem left attached.

- Berries must be detached from the plant, although sometimes it is easier to leave a bit of the stem on. For example, hawthorn berries and elderberries disintegrate if you try to pull them off the stems.

- Roots must be cleaned thoroughly with a nail brush, or even a toothbrush, using running water; patted dry with a clean dish cloth; and then chopped into small pieces, 1cm long or less.

DRYING IN THE OVEN

- Line a baking tray with greaseproof paper.

- Spread your herbs in a thin layer – the root pieces need to be in a single layer, with individual bits just touching each other.

- Set the oven temperature to 40°C/104°F. (Only electric ovens are suitable for this method of drying. Ideally, don't use a fan oven.)

- Timing depends on the herb: the more delicate the plant, the less time it will take to dry. Roughly speaking, leafy plants such as lemon balm take about an hour, while roots and berries take 2-3 hours. You need to check the herbs periodically, and if they look dry and are easily crushed in your fingers they are ready.

STORING DRIED HERBS

There are a number of ways of keeping dried herbs to preserve their medicinal properties. The most important point to remember is to keep them in dry and dark conditions.

- The simplest way is to put your herbs in two brown paper bags, one inside the other. The bags should be folded at the top to the level of the herbs and kept tightly closed with a large paper clip or clothes peg. Keep the bags in a dry cupboard or a drawer.

- Even better, you can put the dry herbs in a paper bag and then put this in another container that can be tightly closed: a tin, glass jar or plastic bag that can be sealed. Such storage gives the herbs the chance to breathe and at the same time minimises the effect of seasonal changes in temperature

and humidity. Keep the container in a dry cupboard or a drawer.

- You can store your herbs in glass or china jars. You should match the amount of herbs to the size of the jar: try to fill the jar to the top and leave a small gap of empty space; if there is a lot of empty space in your container the herbs will lose their fragrance to the air. Also, if the jar is translucent you must keep it away from the light or your herbs will fade in colour and lose their medicinal properties.

- I do not recommend keeping dried herbs directly in a plastic bag unless it is for a short period of time – for instance, if you want to take dry herbs with you on holiday.

SHELF LIFE OF DRY HERBS

- Leaves, flowers, mixed leaves and stems will keep for up to two years, but from time to time check carefully that the colour and smell are not deteriorating. It is also worth checking for any pests: occasionally some eggs or larvae may survive the drying process.

- Roots, seeds, berries will keep for up to four years.

- Some authorities recommend much shorter periods of storage, but, in my experience, if the herbs are stored well their medicinal properties last well too.

Chapter 26
Making your own tinctures, infused oils, syrups and ointments

Caution: Make sure you identify plants correctly before processing, and then label them for storage with the name and date. Keep out of children's reach.

EXTRACT AND PRESERVE

Making your own medicine is great fun and quite easy. The basic principle is that you extract the active constituents from the plant material with a suitable medium and then preserve the product in a suitable way. The medium for extraction is either water, alcohol or oil. The preserving substances are alcohol, oil, sugar, honey or emulsifying ointment (available from chemists). Alcohol and oil act as extracting and preserving substances at the same time.

Below are general instructions for making tinctures, infused oils, syrups and ointments. There are many books that will give you more detailed instructions on making tinctures, especially in terms of alcohol strength and the required period of steeping. However, as we are talking here about small-scale domestic products, the basic instructions given in this chapter will be adequate. In general, fresh herbs make better products, but using dry herbs is quite traditional and perfectly OK too.

MAKING TINCTURES

All the herbs recommended in this book can be made into tinctures using 40% clear vodka or brandy. You can use either fresh herbs or dry ones. If you opt for the fresh herbs your final product will contain a lower percentage of alcohol as the water content of the fresh plant will dilute the alcohol. Each tincture should be made from only a single herb. These can then be used to make specific tincture combinations.

STORAGE

Tinctures should be stored in dark glass bottles with screw-on caps or corks; keep them away from light and heat. Sterilise the bottles before use.

SHELF LIFE

The shelf life of tinctures is, on average, 3-5 years.

HERB-TO-ALCOHOL RATIO

The crucial point about making a tincture is to preserve the right proportion of herbs to alcohol. The herb-to-alcohol ratio, called tincture strength, is expressed in numbers, e.g. 1:2, 1:5, 1:10, etc., where the first number refers to the amount of herbs and the second to the amount of alcohol used in making the tincture (1 part herbs to 2, 5 or 10 parts alcohol). Most of the tinctures referred to in this book are 1:2 strength, which means that you take one part of herbs (in weight) and mix it with 2 parts of alcohol (in weight or volume). For instance, if you have 100g of herbs you will need 200ml (or 200g) of alcohol (for the sake of simplicity you can assume that 1ml and 1g of alcohol are equivalent). Please refer to individual herb descriptions to check the correct tincture strength.

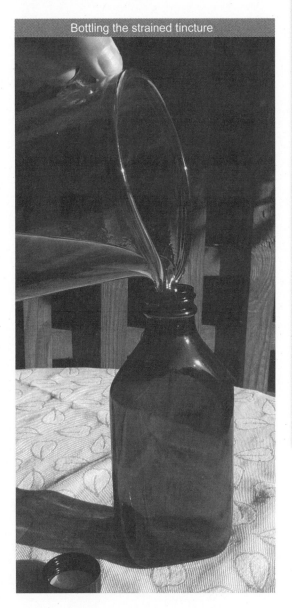

Bottling the strained tincture

TO MAKE A TINCTURE

- Weigh the herbs if you are using dry ones.
- If using fresh herbs, prepare them by chopping them into small pieces, and then weigh them.
- Put the herbs in a large sterilised glass jar with a screw-on top – jars normally used for keeping preserves are fine.
- Measure the right amount of vodka or brandy in a measuring jug.
- Pour the alcohol over the herbs and make sure all the herbs are covered with alcohol; if necessary press the herbs down with a clean spoon.
- Screw the top on and give the jar a good shake.
- Leave to macerate for 2 weeks in a dark place, shaking the jar vigorously every few days.
- Strain the herbs through a jelly bag or cheesecloth, and squeeze them manually to extract all the liquid. You can use a wine press for straining if you have one; the used-up herbs can be composted.
- Poor into dark glass bottles and label with the name of the herb, the tincture strength, the dosage and the date.

MAKING INFUSED OILS

Infused oils can be used on their own for external applications or can be added to various creams or ointments. You can use any good-quality organic oil: sunflower oil or olive oil is used most often. You can use fresh or dry herbs. The herbs most often used for infused oils are: calendula (petals), comfrey (leaf) and St John's wort (flowers).

STORAGE

Infused oils should be stored in dark glass bottles with screw-on caps, away from light and heat.

SHELF LIFE

Store the infused oil in dark glass bottles for up to 2 years.

> ### TO MAKE AN INFUSED OIL
>
> - Prepare fresh herbs by stripping the petals (calendula), chopping the leaves (comfrey) or cutting the flowers off (St John's wort).
> - Fill a sterilised glass jar as tightly as possible with the herbs.
> - Pour the oil in slowly until all the herbs are covered, and screw the top on.
> - Put on a sunny windowsill to infuse for 3-4 weeks; shake the jar occasionally.
> - Strain through a jelly bag or wine press into a jug.
> - Pour into a sterilised dark glass bottle.
> - Label the contents with the name and date of making.

MAKING OINTMENTS

Ointments can be made in a variety of ways, but I have found the recipe below the easiest to use. You can use fresh or dry herbs, and the other ingredients can be bought from a chemist. You can use a variety of herbs, the most common being calendula or comfrey leaf.

SHELF LIFE

Store in dark glass jars for up to 2 years.

> ### TO MAKE AN OINTMENT
>
> - Prepare the herbs: weigh the dry ones or chop the fresh ones and weigh them (if using calendula, strip the petals off the flowers and weigh them).
> - Melt 600g of emulsifying ointment in a glass dish that has been placed in a saucepan half-filled with water on a low heat (emulsifying ointment is a ready-made ointment base available from the chemist).
> - Add 270ml glycerol (available from the chemist).
> - Add 330ml water.
> - Add 120g herbs.
> - Simmer for 3 hours while stirring occasionally, refilling the saucepan with water if necessary.
> - Strain through a jelly bag into a glass bowl while still hot. (Be very careful!)
> - Stir continually until cold.
> - Put into sterilised dark glass jars with a palette knife, making sure that no air pockets are left.
> - Label the contents with the name and date of making.

MAKING SYRUPS

Syrups are the best way to administer cough medicine. Typical herbs used for making syrups are liquorice, thyme, marshmallow root, rose, mullein and hyssop. You can use either dry or fresh herbs or a mixture of the two. I recommend using a single herb per syrup, apart from thyme and liquorice where you can mix the herbs half-and-half.

STORAGE

Syrups should be kept in dark glass bottles, away from light and heat. Syrups made with honey may occasionally ferment: keep the bottle sealed with a cork to prevent an explosion!

SHELF LIFE

Syrups can be kept for 2-3 years.

TO MAKE A HERBAL SYRUP

- Prepare 500ml of a suitable infusion or decoction using 25g of dry herbs or 75g of fresh herbs per 500ml of water.
- Strain the herbs into a saucepan through a cheesecloth and add 500g of honey or unrefined sugar; mix well until the honey/sugar is dissolved.
- Simmer on a low heat, stirring all the time until the syrup thickens.
- Leave to cool down, pour into sterilised glass bottles – do not overfill – and use corks to seal the bottles.
- Label the contents with the name, dosage and date of making.

Part Five
Herbal first-aid kits for travelling

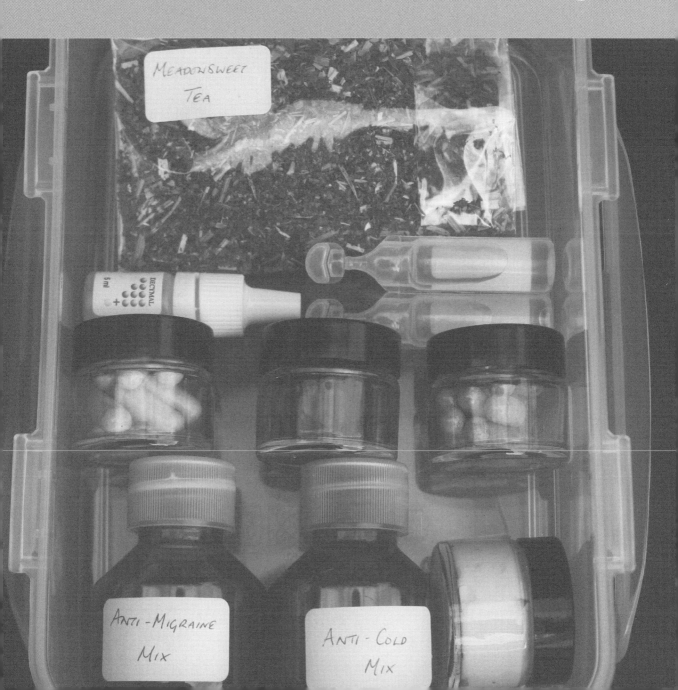

My first-aid kit for travelling consists entirely of herbal products, except for plasters and bandages. It is perhaps a little more bulky than an ordinary first-aid kit because I choose to take herbal liquids. However, good-quality tablets and capsules are perfectly adequate substitutes for tinctures if you are short of space or have weight restrictions.

Liquids need to be carried in your main luggage if you are flying, owing to current anti-terrorist safety measures, although small amounts are permitted in hand luggage. To be sure, check out the regulations when you book your ticket.

You will need to customise your own kit depending on what your common health problems are, and also to include conventional medicines if necessary.

It is important to realise that crossing some international borders with plant products can be an issue, irrespective of whether you go by plane, train, boat or car. Some authorities in countries with a lot of drug problems can be suspicious of anything that doesn't look like conventional medicine. A few countries, for example Australia, ban outright the bringing in of any raw plant products, which would include dry herbs. In general, travelling anywhere in Europe with herbs in any form in your luggage is not a problem; just make sure they are labelled. Beware of taking alcoholic tinctures to some Muslim countries, and on the whole you are on safer ground with tablets rather than tinctures, especially if you have an unopened container. Creams and essential oils should be fine everywhere.

In order to avoid any trouble, please check the restrictions in individual countries and with individual airlines before you go.

Chapter 27
Travelling in Western countries

This basic first-aid kit consists of herbs for travelling in countries with easy access to medical care. I recommend that you keep all the items in a plastic sealable box, so your clothes won't get ruined if one of the bottles leaks. Also, for the purposes of travelling, PET (polyethylene terephthalate) plastic bottles are better than glass; you can get them from the chemist or order them online.

The amount of herbs you will need to take depends on how long you go away for, but for an average holiday you will need 5-10ml of each cream, 50-100ml of each tincture or 3-4 days' worth of herbal tablets.

If there is any ailment that you frequently suffer from, include the herbal treatment for it in your first-aid kit: for example, a cystitis mix or a migraine mix. I don't bother with any special disinfecting herbs as any tincture will do for that purpose, owing to the alcohol content.

Remember that garlic makes great medicine for all sorts of problems and you can get it everywhere. Many countries have a good choice of herbs in their chemists or even supermarkets: for instance, in France and Germany you can always get a wide selection of medicinal herbal teas. Also try to use fresh, locally available herbs such as peppermint and lemon balm.

BASIC FIRST-AID KIT

- 10-20g arnica cream – for bruising, sprains, and tired muscles and joints.

- 10-20g calendula ointment – for sunburn, cuts and small wounds, blisters, insect bites, skin rashes and fungal infections.

- 50 tablets charcoal (they go quickly if you need them) – for any food poisoning, diarrhoea, vomiting or continuing indigestion.

- 60g marshmallow root powder or a capsule equivalent – for heartburn, indigestion, food poisoning and drawing out splinters.

- 100ml anti-diarrhoea mix – for any diarrhoea and food poisoning, and as an insect-bite lotion (see page 58).

- 100ml anti-cold mix made up from 50ml elderflower tincture and 50ml garlic juice – for colds and flu, or a sore throat (winter item).

- 20 propolis capsules – to act as a natural antibiotic.

- 20 propolis lozenges – for a sore throat, together with anti-cold mix or elderflower tea (winter item).

- 50g elderflower tea – as an optional winter item, to prevent or treat colds and flu.

- 50g meadowsweet tea – as an optional item for any digestive problems; include it if you are prone to such problems.

- 100ml thyme-and-liquorice syrup as an optional item; remember that you can always make your own onion syrup (see page 98); I would include it only if you already have a cough or are very prone to getting one (winter item).

- 30 willow tablets – as an optional item to act as a general painkiller and anti-inflammatory; useful if you are prone to a bad back or painful joints.

- 50ml valerian tincture – as an optional item; useful if you get nervous about travelling or if you have any mishap on your holidays.

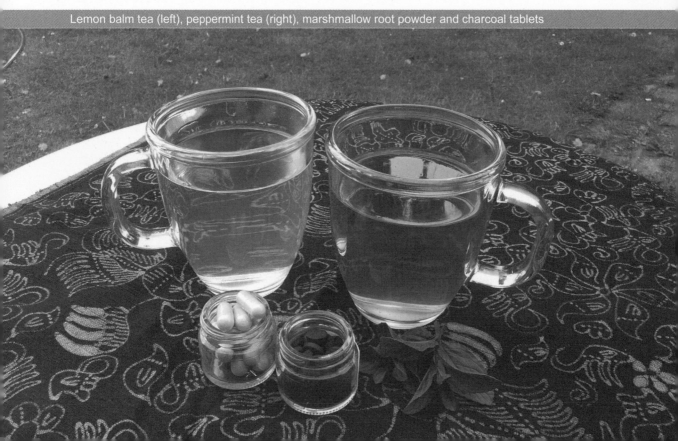

Lemon balm tea (left), peppermint tea (right), marshmallow root powder and charcoal tablets

Chapter 28
Travelling in remote and exotic places

A slightly different selection is needed if you are travelling in countries without easy access to medical care. Your first-aid kit should be versatile and light, containing a small selection of preparations with a multitude of uses suitable for treating typical problems affecting travellers in exotic countries. I recommend taking either tincture mixes or powder capsules of these herbs. Your herbal first-aid kit should match your specific needs, depending on where you are going and what you will be doing.

MALARIA AND HERBS

Herbs can offer only a supportive treatment, not a cure, for many tropical diseases. Unless you are medically qualified it is risky to rely on herbs to treat malaria – different strands often need different treatments. Some people claim that if you use enough insect repellents you won't get bitten by mosquitoes, but such a method is never foolproof, and you only need one bite to contract malaria. You should take precautions to minimise the risk of being infected, but you should also either take the orthodox prophylactics or have conventional treatment available with you (the most effective treatment is still based on plant constituents – quinine and artemisinin). It is a good idea to take milk thistle capsules while taking anti-malarial prophylactics or when you finish the course – milk thistle has a protective action in the liver against some side effects.

PARASITES

You should also exercise great care with food and hygiene to prevent getting infected with parasites – eat only well-cooked food, no salads, peel the fruit, use iodine or chlorine to purify the water, etc. Some parasites from the tropics, for instance giardia, can be successfully treated with herbs, but the treatment is often specific to the parasite so you should seek help when you come back. For the general preventative treatment of digestive problems see Chapter 11, pages 46 and 47.

I recommend that you take larger amounts of specific herbs for those situations when you need a vigorous and prompt treatment, for instance a severe chest infection, severe diarrhoea or an infected wound; the medicine should last you long enough before you reach medical help.

Also take rehydrating salts (supportive treatment for diarrhoea) and sterile saline for treating eye infections and cleaning wounds.

FIRST-AID KIT FOR TRAVELLING IN REMOTE AREAS

- 50g arnica and comfrey cream, mixed half-and-half – for bruising, sprains, tired muscles and joints, head injuries, or broken ribs, toes or fingers.

- 50g calendula ointment – for sunburn, cuts and small wounds, blisters, insect bites, skin rashes, fungal infections, ulcers (including tropical ulcers), sores or bunions.

- 100 charcoal tablets – for food poisoning, diarrhoea, vomiting or continuing indigestion.

- 200ml anti-diarrhoea mix (see page 58) – for diarrhoea and food poisoning and for possible parasitic infection; this can also be used as a lotion for itchy insect bites. It may be more practical to have the same herbs powdered, mixed and put in capsule form: approach your local herbalist if you want to get such capsules.

- 100 propolis capsules – to act as a natural antibiotic for any infection .

- 20ml eyebright tincture in a dropper bottle – to be used with a sterile saline for eye infections, see page 124.

- 20ml tea tree essential oil – for disinfecting cuts, wounds, sores, etc. Use neat, or dilute with clean water or sterile saline.

- 100ml or more of insect repellent – see box.

- 100ml ginkgo tincture (or tablet equivalent) – as an optional item when travelling in a cold climate or at high altitude, to minimise the risk of frostbite or altitude sickness.

HOME-MADE INSECT REPELLENT

Ingredients
- 10-20 drops essential oil of citronella
- 10-20 drops essential oil of lemon-grass or rosemary
- 100ml lavender aromatic water base

To make
- Mix ingredients together and pour into a spray-top container.

Adults and children over 3 years: spray every 4 hours on exposed areas of skin.

Note: not suitable for children under 3 years or for pregnant women.

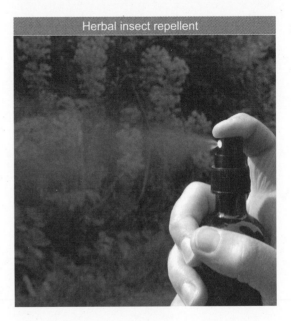
Herbal insect repellent

Appendix 1
Common and Latin herb names

Most of these common herbs can be grown in the UK. Their harvest times, unless otherwise stated, are for the UK.

Aniseed
Botanical name: *Pimpinella anisum*
Part used: seed
Harvest time: when seeds are ripe

Arnica
Botanical name: *Arnica montana*
Part used: flower
Harvest time: when flowers are fully open

Ashwaganda
Botanical name: *Withania somnifera*
Part used: root
Harvest time: late summer

Barberry
Botanical name: *Berberis vulgaris*
Part used: root and/or stem bark
Harvest time: autumn

Bilberries/Blueberries
Botanical name: *Vaccinium myrtillus*
Part used: fruit
Harvest time: summer, when ripe

Birch
Botanical name: *Betula pendula* and *Betula alba*
Part used: leaves, buds
Harvest time: May–July, spring

Black cohosh
Botanical name: *Cimicifuga racemosa*
Part used: root and rhizome
Harvest time: autumn

Celery seed
Botanical name: *Apium graveolens*
Part used: fruit
Harvest time: when ripe

Chamomile (German)
Botanical name: *Matricaria recutita*; *Chamomilla recutita*
Part used: flower
Harvest time: June–August

Chillies (Cayenne pepper)
Botanical name: *Capsicum annuum*
Part used: fruit
Harvest time: when fully ripe (grown in tropical regions)

Comfrey leaf
Botanical name: *Symphytum officinale folium*
Part used: leaf
Harvest time: spring–summer; avoid first leaves and after early October

Couch grass
Botanical name: *Elymus repens*; *Agropyron repens*
Part used: rhizome
Harvest time: March–May or September–October

Cramp bark
Botanical name: *Viburnum opulus*
Part used: bark
Harvest time: no critical time

Damiana
Botanical name: *Turnera diffusa*; *Turnera aphrodisiaca*
Part used: leaf
Harvest time: when flowering (grows in hot and humid climates)

Dandelion leaf
Botanical name: *Taraxacum officinale folium*
Part used: leaf
Harvest time: April–May

Dandelion root
Botanical name: *Taraxacum officinale radix*
Part used: root
Harvest time: autumn

Echinacea (purple coneflower)
Botanical name: *Echinacea angustifolia* and *Echinacea purpurea*
Part used: root
Harvest time: autumn

Elderflower
Botanical name: *Sambucus nigra*
Part used: flower
Harvest time: May–June

Elecampane
Botanical name: *Inula helenium*
Part used: root and rhizome
Harvest time: spring and autumn

Evening primrose
Botanical name: *Oenothera biennis*
Part used: pressed oil from the seed
Harvest time: when ripe, usually September

Eyebright
Botanical name: *Euphrasia* species
Part used: aerial parts
Harvest time: July–September

Fennel
Botanical name: *Foeniculum vulgare*
Part used: leaves, fruit
Harvest time: leaves in summer, fruit in September–October

Garlic
Botanical name: *Allium sativum*
Part used: bulb (cloves)
Harvest time: August

Ginger
Botanical name: *Zingiber officinale*
Part used: rhizome
Harvest time: when plants are 10 months old (grown in tropical regions)

Ginkgo
Botanical name: *Ginkgo biloba*
Part used: leaf
Harvest time: early summer

Green tea
Botanical name: *Camellia sinensis*
Part used: leaf
Harvest time: when leaves are young (grown mainly in Asia)

Ground ivy
Botanical name: *Glechoma hederacea*
Part used: leaves and flowering tops
Harvest time: May

Hawthorn
Botanical name: *Crataegus monogyna* and *Crataegus laevigata*
Part used: leaves with flowers or berries
Harvest time: May–June or September–October

Hops
Botanical name: *Humulus lupulus*
Part used: strobile (fruit)
Harvest time: August–September

Horse chestnut
Botanical name: *Aesculus hippocastanum*
Part used: seed
Harvest time: September

Lavender
Botanical name: *Lavandula officinalis* and *Lavandula angustifolia*
Part used: flower
Harvest time: June–August

Lemon balm
Botanical name: *Melissa officinalis*
Part used: aerial parts
Harvest time: May–October (before flowering)

Lime tree flower
Botanical name: *Tilia cordata*, *Tilia platyphyllos*
and *Tilia* x *europaea*
Part used: flower
Harvest time: early in flowering

Linseed
Botanical name: *Linum usitatissimum*
Part used: seed
Harvest time: September

Liquorice (licorice)
Botanical name: *Glycyrrhiza glabra*
Part used: root
Harvest time: late autumn, when plants are 3-4
years old (grown in southern Europe)

Marigold (calendula)
Botanical name: *Calendula officinalis*
Part used: flower petals
Harvest time: in full flower, in the middle of the day,
June–September

Marshmallow leaf
Botanical name: *Althaea officinalis folium*
Part used: leaf
Harvest time: June

Marshmallow root
Botanical name: *Althaea officinalis radix*
Part used: root (from 2-or-more-year-old plants)
Harvest time: early autumn

Meadowsweet
Botanical name: *Filipendula ulmaria*
Part used: aerial parts
Harvest time: June–July (early in flowering period)

Milk thistle (St Mary's thistle)
Botanical name: *Silybum marianum*
Part used: seed
Harvest time: when ripe

Mountain grape (Oregon grape)
Botanical name: *Berberis aquifolium*; *Mahonia aquifolium*
Part used: root and rhizome
Harvest time: autumn

Nettle leaf
Botanical name: *Urtica dioica folium*
Part used: leaf
Harvest time: May–June

Oats
Botanical name: *Avena sativa*
Part used: green aerial parts
Harvest time: before seeds ripen

Onion
Botanical name: *Allium cepa*
Part used: bulb
Harvest time: autumn

Passionflower
Botanical name: *Passiflora incarnata*
Part used: aerial parts
Harvest time: when flowering (grows in hot, sunny
countries)

Peppermint
Botanical name: *Mentha* x *piperita*
Part used: leaf
Harvest time: May–September

Raspberry leaf
Botanical name: *Rubus idaeus folium*
Part used: leaf
Harvest time: August–September

Red clover
Botanical name: *Trifolium pratense*
Part used: flower
Harvest time: when flowering, in summer

Ribwort plantain
Botanical name: *Plantago lanceolata*
Part used: leaf
Harvest time: during flowering, in May

Rose
Botanical name: *Rosa damascena*, *Rosa gallica* and
Rosa centifolia
Part used: petals from newly opened flowers
Harvest time: June–July

Rosemary
Botanical name: *Rosmarinus officinalis*
Part used: leaf, young twigs
Harvest time: March–October

St John's wort
Botanical name: *Hypericum perforatum*
Part used: aerial parts
Harvest time: during flowering

Sage
Botanical name: *Salvia officinalis*
Part used: leaves
Harvest time: just before flowering

Saw palmetto
Botanical name: *Serenoa repens*; *Serenoa serrulata*
Part used: fruit
Harvest time: autumn (grows in North America)

Shepherd's purse
Botanical name: *Capsella bursa-pastoris*
Part used: aerial parts
Harvest time: April–June

Siberian ginseng
Botanical name: *Eleutherococcus senticosus*
Part used: root
Harvest time: autumn (grows in eastern Russia, China, Korea and Japan)

Tea tree
Botanical name: *Melaleuca alternifolia*
Part used: leaves
Harvest time: all year round (grows in Australia)

Thyme
Botanical name: *Thymus vulgaris*
Part used: leaf and flower
Harvest time: April–September

Turmeric
Botanical name: *Curcuma longa*
Part used: rhizome
Harvest time: winter (grown in South Asia)

Valerian
Botanical name: *Valeriana officinalis*
Part used: root and rhizome
Harvest time: September–October

Vervain
Botanical name: *Verbena officinalis*
Part used: aerial parts
Harvest time: early stages of flowering

White deadnettle
Botanical name: *Lamium album*
Part used: flowering tops
Harvest time: April–July

Wild yam
Botanical name: *Dioscorea villosa*
Part used: rhizome
Harvest time: autumn (grown in sunny regions, both tropical and temperate)

Willow bark
Botanical name: *Salix alba* and *Salix purpurea*
Part used: bark from 2-5-year-old trees
Harvest time: April–May

Wintergreen
Botanical name: *Gaultheria procumbens*
Part used: leaves
Harvest time: leaves may be collected at any time (for essential oil only)

Witch hazel
Botanical name: *Hamamelis virginiana*
Part used: leaf, bark
Harvest time: autumn

Yarrow
Botanical name: *Achillea millefolium*
Part used: aerial parts
Harvest time: in full flower

Yellow dock (curled dock)
Botanical name: *Rumex crispus*
Part used: root
Harvest time: October

Appendix 2
Glossary of actions

Adaptogen – a substance that helps the body cope with stress, either physical or mental

Adrenal tonic – a substance that improves the function of the adrenal glands

Anaesthetic – a substance that brings about a reversible loss of consciousness

Analgesic – a substance that relieves pain

Antacid – a substance that neutralises acidity in the stomach

Anti-allergic – a substance that reduces the intensity or frequency of allergic reactions

Anti-arthritic – a substance that reduces joint inflammation

Antibacterial – a substance that destroys bacteria or inhibits bacterial growth

Anti-catarrhal – a substance that reduces the production of catarrh or phlegm

Anti-coagulant – a substance that prevents the formation of blood clots

Antidepressant – a substance that alleviates depression

Anti-diarrhoeal – a substance that stops diarrhoea

Anti-fungal – a substance that destroys fungi or inhibits fungal growth

Anti-inflammatory – a substance that reduces inflammation

Anti-irritant – a substance that reduces local surface inflammation (internal or external)

Antimicrobial – a substance that destroys microorganisms or inhibits the growth of microorganisms (this term is usually used when referring to internal use; cf. 'Antiseptic', below)

Antioxidant – a substance that is capable of slowing or preventing the damaging effects of oxidation and free radicals

Anti-platelet – a substance that reduces the clumping together of platelets – small blood cells that play a part in the formation of blood clots

Anti-rheumatic – a substance that alleviates rheumatic complaints

Antiseptic – a substance that destroys microorganisms or inhibits their growth (this term is usually used when referring to external use; cf. 'Antimicrobial', above)

Antiviral – a substance that inhibits virus replication or destroys viruses

Aphrodisiac – a substance that stimulates sex drive

Astringent – a substance that causes shrinkage of mucous membranes or exposed tissues, thus creating a surface barrier

Bitter (tonic) – a substance that tastes bitter and stimulates the whole of the digestive system through its bitter taste in the mouth

Carminative – a substance that alleviates flatulence (excessive gas) and relieves bowel spasm

Circulatory stimulant – a substance that improves the circulation of blood, either to particular parts of the body or to all tissues

Cooling – a substance that reduces the sensation of feeling hot, either of a particular body part or of the whole body

Demulcent – a substance that reduces irritation and has a soothing effect on the mucous membranes of the digestive, respiratory and urinary systems

Detoxifying – a substance that improves the elimination of metabolic waste from the body (the terms 'depurative', 'blood purifying' or 'alterative' have been used in the past)

Digestive – a substance that improves or stimulates the digestion

Disinfectant – a substance that is capable of destroying microorganisms on contact; in connection with living tissue the term 'antiseptic' is normally used

Diuretic – a substance that increases the production of urine

Expectorant – a substance that improves the clearing of excess mucus from the airways

Healing – a substance that stimulates tissue repair

Immune modulator – a substance that balances the functioning of the immune system

Immune stimulant – a substance that stimulates the activity of a particular set of immune system cells

Laxative – a substance that induces bowel movement or loosens the stool

Male tonic – a substance that improves the function of the male reproductive system

Mucous membrane restorative – a substance that facilitates the repair of damaged or inflamed mucous membrane

Relaxant (muscles) – a substance that decreases the tone of muscles, especially if the muscles are in spasm

Relaxant (nerves) – a substance that has a calming effect on the nervous system

Restorative – a substance that restores optimal function to a body organ or tissue

Sedative – a substance that reduces nervous tension, which is used to relieve anxiety or induce sleep

Stimulant – a substance that increases the activity of a particular organ or system or the whole body

Tonic – a substance that improves the function and vigour of a particular organ or system or the whole body

Warming – a substance that increases the sensation of feeling warm, either of a particular body part or of the whole body

References

1   Anghelescu, I. G., Kohnen, R., Szegedi, A., Klement, S. & Kieser, M. (2006). 'Comparison of Hypericum extract WS 5570 and paroxetine in ongoing treatment after recovery from an episode of moderate to severe depression: results from a randomized multicenter study'. *Pharmacopsychiatry*, Nov 2006; 39(6): 213-19.

Brenner, R., Azbel, V., Madhusoodanan, S. & Pawlowska, M. (2000). 'Comparison of an extract of Hypericum (LI 160) and sertraline in the treatment of depression: a double-blind, randomized pilot study'. *Comp Clin Ther*, Apr 2000; 22(4): 411-19.

Gastpar, M., Singer, A. & Zeller, K. (2006). 'Comparative efficacy and safety of a once-daily dosage of Hypericum extract STW3-VI and citalopram in patients with moderate depression: a double-blind, randomised, multicentre, placebo-controlled study'. *Pharmacopsychiatry*, Mar 2006; 39(2): 66-75.

Schrader, E. (2000). 'Equivalence of St John's wort extract (Ze 117) and fluoxetine: a randomized, controlled study in mild-moderate depression'. *Int Clin Psychopharmacol*, Mar 2000; 15(2): 61-8.

2   Zakay-Rones, Z., Thom, E., Wollan, T. & Wadstein, J. (2004). 'Randomized study of the efficacy and safety of oral elderberry extract in the treatment of influenza A and B virus infections'. *J Int Med Res*, Mar–Apr 2004; 32(2): 132-40.

Zakay-Rones, Z., Varsano, N., Zlotnik, M., Manor, O., Regev, L., Schlesinger, M. & Mumcuoglu, M. (1995). 'Inhibition of several strains of influenza virus in vitro and reduction of symptoms by an elderberry extract Sambucus nigra during an outbreak of influenza B Panama'. *J Altern Complement Med*, Winter 1995; 1(4): 361-9.

3   Hopkins, A.B. (2003). 'Chicken soup cure may not be a myth'. *Nurse Pract*, Jun 2003; 28(6): 16.

Jackson, P.M. (1994). 'Chicken soup'. *Wis Med J*, Jan 1994; 93(1): 3.

Jefferson, T. (2002). 'Advances in the diagnosis and management of influenza'. *Curr Infect Dis Rep*, Jun 2002; 4(3): 206-10.

Ohry, A. & Tsafrir, J. (1999). 'Is chicken soup an essential drug?'. *CMAJ*, Dec 1999; 161(12): 1532-3.

Rennard, B.O., Ertl, R.F., Gossman, G.L., Robbins, R.A. & Rennard, S.I. (2000). 'Chicken soup inhibits neutrophil chemotaxis in vitro'. *Chest*, 118(4): 1150-7.

Saketkhoo, K., Januszkiewicz, A. & Sackner, M.A. (1978). 'Effect of drinking hot water, cold water, and chicken soup on nasal mucus velocity and nasal airflow resistance'. *Chest*, Oct 1978; 74(4): 408-10.

4   Mathias, A. et al. (2004). 'The caco-2 intestinal absorption model of Echinacea Premium extract'. *J Clin Pharm Ther*, 29: 7-13.

Mathias, A. et al. (2005). 'Bioavailability of Echinacea constituents: Caco-2 monolayers and pharmacokinetics of the alkylamides and caffeic acid conjugates'. *Molecules*, 10: 1242-51.

Miller, S.C. (2005). 'Echinacea: a miracle herb against aging and cancer? Evidence *in vivo* in mice'. eCAM 2(3): 309-14. www.mediherb.com.au/articles (links and articles on *Echinacea* species).

Raduner, S., Majewska, A., Chen, J.Z. et al. (2006). 'Alkylamides from Echinacea are a new class of cannabinomimetics'. *J Biol Chem*, 281(2): 14192-206.

Shah, S.A., Sander, S., White, C.M., Rinaldi, M. & Coleman, C.I. (2007). 'Evaluation of Echinacea for the prevention and treatment of the common cold: a meta-analysis'. *Lancet Infect Dis*, Jul 2007; 7(7): 473-80.

Stevenson, L.M. et al. (2005). 'Modulation of the immune responses of macrophages by Echinacea alkyl amides'. *Molecules*, 10: 1279-85.

5   Beasley, R., Clayton, T., Crane, J., von Mutius, E., Lai, C.K. & Montefort, S. (2008). 'Association between paracetamol use in infancy and childhood, and risk of asthma, rhinoconjunctivitis, and eczema in children aged 6-7 years: analysis from Phase Three of the ISAAC programme'. *The Lancet*, 372(9643): 1039-48.

6   Barak, V., Birkenfeld, S., Halperin, T. & Kalickman, I. (2002). 'The effect of herbal remedies on the production of human inflammatory and anti-inflammatory cytokines'. *Isr Med Assoc J*, Nov 2002; 4(11 Suppl): 919-22.

Sun, J., Madan, R., Karp, C.L. & Braciale, T.J. (2009). 'Effector T cells control lung inflammation during acute influenza virus infection by producing IL-10'. *Nat Med*, Mar 2009; 15(3): 277-84. Epub 22 Feb 2009.

Zambon, M.C. (2001). 'The pathogenesis of influenza in humans'. *Rev Med Virol*, Jul–Aug 2001; 11(4): 227-41.

Zhai, Z., Liu, Y., Wu, L., Senchina, D.S., Wurtele, E.S., Murphy, P.A., Kohut, M.L. & Cunnick, J.E. (2007). 'Enhancement of innate and adaptive immune functions by multiple *Echinacea* species'. *J Med Food*, Sep 2007; 10(3): 423-34.

Bibliography

BOOKS

Barker, J. (2001), *The Medicinal Flora of Britain and Northwest Europe*, Winter Press

Bartram, T. (2002), *Bartram's Encyclopedia of Herbal Medicine*, Da Capo Press

Bone, K. (2007), 'Phytotherapy for anti-aging and Cardiovascular health', Mediherb Seminar, seminar notes May 2007

Bone, K. (2007) *The Ultimate Herbal Compendium*, Phytotherapy Press

Bradley, P. (2006) *British Herbal Compendium Vol 2: A handbook of scientific information on widely used plant drugs*, British Herbal Medical Association

British Herbal Pharmacopeia (1983), British Herbal Medical Association

Mills, S. & Bone, K. (2005) *The Essential Guide to Herbal Safety*, Churchill Livingstone

Mills, S. & Bone, K. (2000) *Principles and Practice of Phytotherapy*, Churchill Livingstone

Ody, P. (1995) *Home Herbal*, Macmillan Canada

Thomsen, M. (2002) *Phytotherapy Desk Reference*, 2nd edn, Institut for Phytotherapi

Trickey, R. & Cooke, K. (2001) *Women's Trouble*, Allen & Unwin

Trickey, R. & Cooke, K. (2002) *Menopause*, Allen & Unwin

RESEARCH PAPERS

Beer, A.M. & Wegener, T. (2008). *Phytomedicine* 15(11): 907-13. (Randomised, double-blind, placebo-controlled clinical study of the effectiveness of willow extract.)

Cui, Y., Shu, X.O., Gao, Y.T. et al. (2006). 'Korean ginseng and breast cancer survival'. *Am J Epidemiol*, 163(7): 645-53.

Daniele, C., Mazzanti, G., Pittler, M.H. et al. (2006). *Drug Safety*, 29(6): 523-35. (Study assessing the safety of hawthorn of 24 clinical studies.)

El-Kamary, S., Shardell, M., Metwally, M. et al. (2007). *Am J Trop Med Hyg*, 77(5): 210. (Randomised, double-blind, placebo-controlled clinical study on the efficacy of milk thistle in recovery from acute hepatitis.)

Holubarsch, C.J., Colucci, W.S., Meinertz, T. et al. (2008). *Eur J Heart Fail*, 10(12): 1255-63. (Randomised, double-blind, placebo-controlled study of the effectiveness of hawthorn in heart failure patients.)

Koo, H., Gomes, B.P., Rosalen, P.L., Ambrosano, G.M., Park, Y.K. & Cury, J.A. (2000). 'In vitro antimicrobial activity of propolis and Arnica Montana against oral pathogens'. *Arch Oral Biol*, Feb 2000; 45(2): 141-8.

Muller, S.F. & Klement, S. (2006). 'Uncontrolled study of valerian/lemon balm for the treatment of restlessness and dyssomnia in children'. *Phytomedicine*, 13(6): 383-7.

Ozan, F., Sümer, Z., Polat, Z.A., Er, K., Ozan, U. & Değer, O. (2007). 'Effects of mouth rinse containing propolis on oral microorganisms and human gingival fibroblasts'. *Eur J Dent*, Oct 2007; 1(4): 195-201.

Paulsen, E. (2002). 'Contact sensitization from *Compositae*-containing herbal remedies and cosmetics'. *Contact Dermatitis*, Oct 2002; 47(4): 189-98.

Rouhi, H. & Ganji, F. (2007). *Pakistan J Nutr*, 6(3): 256-8. (Randomised, double-blind, placebo-controlled clinical study on the effectiveness of marshmallow extract and ACE inhibitor cough.)

Sobenin, I.A., Andrianova, I.V., Demidova, O.N. et al. (2008). *J Atheroscler Thromb*, 15(6): 334-8. (Randomised, double-blind, placebo-controlled clinical study for the lipid-lowering effects of garlic powder tablets.)

Suh, S.O, Kroh, M., Kim, N.R. et al. (2002) 'Korean ginseng and survival of the patients with gastric carcinoma'. *Am J Chin Med*, 30(4): 483-94.

Teschke, R. & Schwarzenboek, A. (2009). 'Critical analysis of suspected adverse reactions to *Cimicifuga racemosa*'. *Phytomedicine*, 16(1): 72-84.

WEBSITES

www.bmj.com (medical research)

www.nature.com (scientific and medical papers)

www.ncbi.nlm.nih.gov (a free digital archive of biomedical and life sciences journal literature)

www.thelancet.com (scientific and medical papers)

Resources

UK-BASED RETAILERS; MAIL-ORDER SUPPLIERS OF HERBS; TRADE & PRACTITIONER SUPPLIERS

Avicenna (high-quality herbal tinctures; large selection of aromatic waters; sales to practitioners only)
Bidarren, Cilcennin
Lampeter, Ceredigion
Wales SA48 8RL ☎ 01570 471000
www.avicennaherbs.co.uk

BeeVital (high-quality propolis products online)
Nature's Laboratory Ltd (UK distributor)
Brereton Lodge
Goathland, Whitby
North Yorks YO22 5JR ☎ 01947 602346
www.beevitalpropolis.com

Culpeper UK Ltd (a niche retail company selling herbal products, natural skincare and aromatherapy oils)
Mail order: ☎ 01451 822681
www.culpeper.co.uk

G. Baldwin & Co (large selection of good-quality herbal products; sales online and through catalogue)
171/173 Walworth Road
London SE17 1RW ☎ 020 7703 5550
www.baldwins.co.uk

Granary Herbs Ltd (specialist in high-quality tinctures made from fresh native herbs; sales mainly to herbalists)
The Granary
Milgate Park, Bearsted
Kent ME14 4NN ☎ 01622 739781
www.granaryherbs.co.uk

Lamberts Healthcare Ltd (good-quality herbal tablets and capsules; sales to health professionals)
1 Lamberts Road
Tunbridge Wells
Kent TN2 3EH ☎ 01892 554314
www.lambertshealthcare.co.uk

Mediherb Pty Ltd (the highest-quality herbal tinctures and tablets; sales to practitioners only)
Balance Healthcare Ltd (UK distributor)
7-10 Langston Priory Mews
Station Road, Kingham
Oxfordshire OX7 6UP ☎ 01608 658862
www.mediherb.co.uk

Neal's Yard Remedies (a chain of retailers selling herbal products and natural cosmetics; branches in most UK cities; online shop)
Mail order: ☎ 01747 834698
www.nealsyardremedies.com

Organic Herb Trading Company (wide range of organically sourced herbs; suppliers to practitioners and retail)
Milverton, Somerset TA4 1NF ☎ 01823 401205
www.organicherbtrading.com

Phyto Products Ltd
Park Works, Park Road
Mansfield Woodhouse
Nottinghamshire NG19 8EF ☎ 01623 644334
Email: info@phyto.co.uk

Proline Botanicals Ltd (wide range of good-quality herbal products; sales to practitioners and retail)
Meadow Park Industrial Estate
Bourne Road, Essendine, nr Stamford
Lincolnshire PE9 4LT ☎ 01780 753366
www.prolinebotanicals.com

Pukka Herbs Ltd (high-quality Ayurvedic herbs; sales to practitioners, clinics and retail outlets)
8 Hawkfield Business Park
Bristol BS14 0BY ☎ 0845 375 1744
www.pukkaherbs.com

Rosa Medica Ltd (amazing-quality essential oils; large selection)
The Barn, Crickham
Wedmore, Somerset BS28 4JT ☎ 01934 712848
www.rosamedica.com

Rutland Biodynamics Ltd (biodynamic growers and manufactures of high-quality and wide range of herbal products; sales to practitioners, clinics and retail)
Unit 21 Langston Priory Mews
Station Road, Kingham
Oxfordshire OX7 6UP ☎ 01608 659600
www.rutlandbio.com

Weleda (UK) Ltd (natural cosmetics; good selection of herbal creams and ointments; catalogue or online sales)
Heanor Road, Ilkeston
Derbyshire DE7 8DR ☎ 0115 944 8222
www.weleda.co.uk

HERB NURSERIES

Arne Herbs (wide selection of medicinal plants)
Limeburn Nurseries, Limeburn Hill
Chew Magna, Bristol BS40 8QW ☎ 01275 333399
www.arneherbs.co.uk

Jekka's Herb Farm (the UK's leading organic herb grower, with a very wide selection of medicinal herbs and seeds)
Rose Cottage, Shellards Lane
Alveston, Bristol BS35 3SY ☎ 01454 418878
www.jekkasherbfarm.com

The National Herb Centre (good selection of medicinal plants)
Banbury Road, Warmington
Warks OX17 1DF ☎ 01295 690999
www.herbcentre.co.uk

Poyntzfield Herb Nursery (good variety of native medicinal herbs, plus unusual Asian species)
Black Isle, By Dingwall
Ross & Cromarty IV7 8LX, Scotland
☎ 01381 610352
www.poyntzfieldherbs.co.uk

ORGANISATIONS AND REGISTERS OF PROFESSIONAL HERBALISTS IN UK

The following represent a European tradition of herbal medicine.

CPP (The College of Practitioners of Phytotherapy, an organisation with a strong scientific and evidence base bias; runs a register of practitioners)
Oak Glade
9 Hythe Close, Polegate
East Sussex BN26 6LQ ☎ 01323 484353
www.phytotherapists.org

NIMH (The National Institute of Medical Herbalists, the oldest herbalist organisation in the UK; runs a register of practitioners)
Elm House
54 Mary Arches Street
Exeter, Devon EX4 3BA ☎ 01392 426022
www.nimh.org.uk

BHMA (British Herbal Medical Association, an organisation fostering research into herbal medicine; members include growers, manufacturers and academics)
PO Box 583
Exeter EX1 9GX ☎ 0845 680 1134
www.bhma.info

The Herb Society (educational charity encouraging the use of herbs)
Sulgrave Manor
Sulgrave, Banbury OX17 2SD ☎ 0845 491 8699
www.herbsociety.co.uk

Index

Page numbers in bold indicate where the fullest information for a herb or ailment may be found.

acne 114, 115, 117, **119-20**
acne rosacea 38, 44, 117, 133
adaptogens 152, 153, 160
adrenal exhaustion 84, 154, 164
ageing process 162-3
allergic reactions to herbs 12, 17
anaemia **39-40**
angina 44, 62
animal self-medication 13
aniseed **50-1**, 59, **185**
ankylosing spondylitis 79
antibacterials 112, 164-5
anti-catarrhals 95, 102, 103
anti-inflammatories 47, 70, 72, 73, 74, 91, 101, 103, 114, 115, 117, 153
anti-virals 11, 91, 95, 103, 110, 164-5
anxiety 13, 39, 48, 53, 81, 83, 85, **86-7**, 93
aphrodisiacs 139
appetite, lack of **56**
arnica 40, **68-9**, 75-6, 79, 156, 157, 181, 183, **185**
arteries, clogged 35, 42, 163
arthritis 70, 73, 79
ashwaganda **153**, 154, 155, 156, 159, 160, 161, 164, 165, **185**
aspirin 13, 70
asthma 112
athlete's foot **121**

back pain 70, 74, **75**, 79
bacteria in the gut 46-7
barberry 28, **51**, 56, 58, 60, 65, 125, 164, 171, **185**
bearberry 20
bedwetting **141**
benign prostatic enlargement **141**

bilberries *see* blueberries
birch **73**, **185**
black cohosh **138-9**, 143, 144, 170, 171, **185**
bleeding
    blood in stools 67
    cuts and small wounds **40**
    nosebleeds 34, **43**
    staunching 35
    bloating 47, 50, 51, **56-7**, 59, 65, 147
blood clot formation 35, 163
blood pressure
    high 12, 35, 36, 37, 38, 39, **41-2**, 44, 163
    low **43**
blue cohosh 20
blueberries/bilberries **36-7**, 41, 43, 143, **162**, **185**
boils 117, **121-2**
breastfeeding women 27
bronchitis 99, **103-4**, 112
bruising 34, **40-1**, 72, **75-6**, 114
bumps and knocks 69
burns 114, **122-3**
buying herbs 167-8

cabbage leaf poultice 76
calendula 41, 59, 61-2, 63, 92, 108, **114**, 120, 123, 125-6, 127, 128, 129, 130, 131-2, 148, 164, 169, 170, 171, 173, 177, 181, 183-4, **187**
cancers 67, 162-3
capsules/tablets 21, 23
car/sea sickness 52
cardiovascular disease 34, 163
catarrh 95, 102, 103, 110
cat's claw 20
cedar 158
celery seed **71**, 76, 77, **139**, 142, **185**
cellulitis 45

chamomile 9, **47-8**, 56, 57, 58, 60, 61, 63, 64, 65, 66, **82**, 87, 89, 91, **114-15**, 119-20, 126, 128, 130, 146, 147, 169, 170, 171, 173, **185**
charcoal 28, **50**, 58, 60, 64, 66, 181, 184
chaste tree 143
chest infections 97, 99, 100, 106
    see also bronchitis; colds; flu
chest pain 45
chicken broth 94-5
chilblains 34, 37, **41**, 43
children
    babies, treating 16, 23, 26
    choosing the right herbs 29
    dosage 26-7
    see also specific remedies and ailments for advice
chillies 36, 37, 41, 43, **72**, 77, **185**
cholesterol, high 35, **42**, 44, 163
chronic fatigue syndrome 55, 112, 154, 164
cinnamon 36, 56, 158
circulation, poor 34, 36, 37, 38, 41, **43-4**
circulatory system 34-45
cold hands and feet 34, 36
cold sores **123**
colds **104-6**
    prevention of 95, 96, 98, **104-5**
    treatment 28, 94, 95, 96, 99, 100, 102, **105-6**
    see also flu
colic **57**
combining herbs 30-1
comfrey **69-70**, 75, 76, 77, 78, 79, **114**, 129, 156, 157, 171, 177, 183, **185**
compresses 23-4
concentration aids 36, 82, **87-8**, 152, 162

coneflower *see* echinacea
conjunctivitis 116, **124**, 134
constipation 53, **57-8**, 119
couch grass **136**, 142, **185**
coughs 97, 99, 100, 101, 104
    dry 102, 104, **106**, 112
    persistent 100, 107, 112
    productive 104, **107**, 112
cradle cap **124-5**
cramp bark **70**, 78, **136**, 141, 146,
    171, **185**
cranberry juice 142
creams and ointments 23
culinary herbs 170
cuts and grazes **40**, 114, 115, **125**,
    134
cystitis 136, 137, **141-2**, 148, 149

damiana **139**, 144, 158, 159, 160,
    161, **185**
dandelion 13, 133, 147, 170, **186**
dandelion root **51-2**, 56, 57, 65,
    128, 172, **186**
dandruff **125-6**
decoctions 22-3
dementia 162
depression 11, 13, 84, 85, **88**, 93, 151
detoxifiers 71, 73, 117, 119
diarrhoea 16, 49, 50, 51, 52, 53,
    54, 55, **58**, 60, 64, 67, 184
digestive stimulants 50, 53, 55
digestive system 46-67
digoxin 13
dill 170
diuretics 13, 71, 95, 136, 138
diverticular disease 49, 53, 67
dosage 15, 16, 25-7
    essential oils 26
    herb mixes 30-1
    length of treatment 27
    older people 27
    teas 25-6
    tinctures 25
    when to take herbs 27
drying herbs 173-4
duodenal ulcers 66

ear infections, recurrent **108**
earache 81, 103, **107-8**
echinacea 12, 18, 20, 92, **98-9**,
104, 105, 106, 108, 109, **115-16**,
122, 125, 131, **137**, 142, **163**, 164,
165, 171, 172, **186**
eczema 59, 114, 115, 116, 117, 119,
    126-8, 130, 133
elderflower 11, 28, **95-6**, 103, 104,
    105, 106, 107, 108, 109, 110,
    111, 123, 164, 169, 170, 171, 173,
    181, **186**
elecampane **100**, 106, 107, 171,
    172, **186**
endometriosis 148
energy
    boosters 152-4
    low 151-2
    see also stamina, mental and
        physical
environmental issues 15, 18-20
    endangered herbs 18, 20
    native/imported herbs 18-19,
        168
    organic cultivation 19, 169
    overharvesting 18
    wild harvesting 19-20
ephedrine 13
erectile dysfuntion **143**
essential oils 23
    in bathwater 26
    carrier oils 26
    dosage 26
    precautions 12, 16, 23, 26
evening primrose 147, 170, 171, **186**
exam nerves 81, **88-9**
extracting and preserving
    substances 175
eye bath 124
eyebright 110, **116**, 124, 132, 171,
    184, **186**
eyes
    itchiness 116
    puffy/tired 116, **129-30**
    sore 115, 124
    watering 116

false unicorn 18, 20
fennel 57, 59, 170, 171, **186**
fevers 16, 101, 105, **108-9**
fibromyalgia 78, 79
first-aid kit 9, 180-4
flu 95, 99, **109-10**

food intolerances **59-60**
food poisoning 50, 51, 52, **60**, 66
fractures 69, **76**
fungal infections 115, 121, 133, 134

gall bladder removal **60-1**
gallstones 57, 67
gargles 63, 102, 111
garlic 28, **35**, 41-2, 42, **52**, 64, 66,
    96-7, 103, 104, 105, 110, 111,
    130-1, 133, 147, **163**, 164, 170,
    186
garlic juice 96, 97, 106, 110, 111, 112
gastritis 49, 51, 53
ginger 36, **37**, 41, 43, **52**, 56, 63,
    105, 156, 158, 160, **186**
ginkgo 36, 41, 43, 44, 156, 158,
    160, 161, **162**, 171, 184, **186**
ginseng
    Korean 18, 20, 43, 92, 144, **153**,
        155, 156, 158, 159, **162-3**
    Siberian 87, 92, 93, **152-3**, 154,
        155, 156, 158, 164, 165, **188**
glands, swollen 112
golden seal 18, 20
gout 71, 73, **76-7**, 79
green tea **163**, **186**
ground ivy **100-1**, 107, 172, **186**
growing herbs 169-72
gum problems **61**

haemorrhoids (piles) 34, 38, **44**,
    55, **61-2**
hair loss 134
hawthorn **37-8**, 41, 44, 143, 144,
    145, 156, 158, 159, 160, **163**,
    169, 170, 171, 173, **186**
hay fever **110**, 112
headaches 45, 79, 93, 112
    migraine 93
    tension headaches 70, 81, **89**
heart attack, recovery from 37
herbal apothecaries 168
herbal medicine
    affordability 8, 13
    bioavailability 12
    biochemical complexity 12-13
    bodily self-healing 12
    combining herbs 30-1
    drugs/herbs interaction 13, 17

effectiveness 11
evidence base 11
matching to the ailment 28-9
non-addictive 13, 80
safety guidelines 16-17
side effects 11-12
symptom assessment 28
unsuccessful treatment 32
see also dosage
herbal shampoos 126
herbs
buying 167-8
culinary 170
drying and storing 173-4
growing 19, 169-72
see also environmental issues
herpes 91
hiatus hernia 47, 48, **62**
holiday digestive problems **64**
honey 94
hops 65, **83**, 87, 90, 91, 126, 171, **186**
horse chestnut **38**, 126, **186**
horseradish 36, 43
hot flushes 137, 139, **143-4**, 145
hyperactivity 81
hypertrophy **141**
hyssop 178

illness, recovering from 164-5
immune system, strengthening
12, 152
impetigo 134
incontinence **144**
indigestion 28, 48, 83, **91**
infertility/low sperm count 148
inflammatory bowel disease 49, 54
infused oils 177
infusions 21, 22, 30
for children 26-7
cold-water infusions 50
diuretics 138
dosage 25-6
herb mixtures 31
making 22
insect bites and stings 114, 115, 184
insect repellent 184
insomnia 13, 85, **90**
iron tonics 39
irritable bowel syndrome (IBS)
48, 49, 53, 54, 56, 66

itchy scalp **125-6**
itchy skin 115, **128**

Jesuit's bark 20
joint inflammation and pain 70,
71, 74, **77-8**, 79
joint recovery (after exercise) 157

kidney stones 136, 148, 149

labdanum 158
lavender **72**, 78, **81-2**, 89, 90, **116-
17**, 157, 170, 171, **186**
leg ulcers 38, 44
lemon balm **53**, 62, 64, **83**, 87, 89,
92, 123, 126, 147, 158, 159, 169,
171, **186**
lemongrass 184
libido
low 139, **144**, 148, 158
reviving 158-9
lime tree flower **38**, 42, **83-4**, 89,
101, 105, 109, 171, **187**
linden *see* lime tree flower
linseed **53**, 57, 60, 122, 163, 171, **187**
liquorice 28, **53-4**, 62, 64, 77, **84**,
93, **101**, 104, 106, 107, **154**, 155,
156, 164, 165, 178, 182, **187**
liver disease 66-7
liver regeneration 54
liver, sluggish 51, 56

malaria 183
marigold *see* calendula
marshmallow leaf **49**, 59, 60,
104, 106, **136**, 141, 142, 144,
171, **187**
marshmallow root 24, **48-9**, 58,
60, 62, 64, 65, 91, **102**, 106,
131, 178, 181, **187**
ME *see* chronic fatigue syndrome
meadowsweet 28, **47**, 62, 65, **72-3**,
169, 171, 182, **187**
memory enhancers 36, 152, 162, 163
menopausal problems 85, 86,
139, 140, 143, **145**, 148
migraine 93
milk thistle **54**, 171, 183, **187**
moles 134
molluscum contagiosum 133

mood swings 55, 85, 86, 139, 145
morning sickness 27, 48, **63**
mountain grape **102**, 106, 112, **117**,
120, 125, 129, 171, **187**
mouth ulcers **63**
mouthwashes 61
mullein 178
multiple sclerosis 93
muscle aches and pains 38, 70,
71, **78**, 79
muscle cramps **78**
muscle recovery (after exercise)
157
muscle strength, rebuilding 153
muscle tension/spasm 70, 71,
72, 73
muscular and skeletal systems
68-79
myrrh 158

nappy rash 114, **128-9**
nausea 52, **63-4**
neck pain 70
nervous exhaustion 84
nervous indigestion 48, **91**
nervous system 80-93
nettle leaf **73**, 76, 77, **117**, 141, 172,
187
see also white deadnettle
neuralgia 85, **91**, 93
nose, blocked/runny 95, **103**, 110
nosebleeds 34, **43**
nutmeg 158
nutrition, healthy 46

oat bath 127
oats **84**, 88, 93, 154, 160, 161, 164,
172, **187**
onion **97**, **187**
onion syrup 97, 98, 104, 106, 107
orchitis 138
osteoarthritis 71, 74, 79

palpitations 39, 44
panic attacks **91-2**
parasites 183
passionflower **85**, 87, 89, 91, 158,
187
pelvic inflammatory disease 149
peppermint **48**, 57, 59, 64, **73**, 78,

169, 170, 171, **187**
peptic ulcer 49, 53
period disorders 35, 55, 138, 148
    heavy periods 38, 140, **145-6,**
      149
    painful periods 81, 136, **146**
poisonous plants 20
polycystic ovary syndrome (PCOS)
    148
post-viral fatigue 95, 164
poultices 24
powdered herbs 23
pregnant women 23, 27, 29
premenstrual syndrome (PMS)
    80, **146-7,** 148
probiotics 46-7, 57, 59
professional help, seeking 14, 16
propolis 28, 61, 63, **99,** 104, 110,
    111, 112, 120, 122, 125, 131, 132,
    164, 165, 181, 184
prostatitis 136
psoriasis 117, 119, **129,** 133
psyllium 57

rashes 114, **130,** 134
raspberry leaf **54-5, 187**
red clover **117,** 120, 129, 172, **187**
reflux (heartburn) 47, 48, 49, 52,
    62, 65
relaxants
    muscles 70, 71, 72, 73, 136
    nerves 38, 39, 53, 81, 83, 86, 118
respiratory system 94-112
restless leg syndrome 79
rheumatoid arthritis 71, 74, 79
ribwort plantain **117-18,** 120, 128,
    129, 130, 170, 172, **187**
rose **85,** 88, 145, 158, 160, 164, 171,
    173, 178, **187**
rosemary **38-9, 71,** 75, 78, **82,** 87-8,
    103, 126, 156, 157, 170, 171, 184,
    188
rutin 40, 43

sage 61, 63, **102-3,** 111, **139-40,**
    143, 144, 145, 170, 171, **188**
St John's wort 11, **85-6,** 88, 91, **103,**
    107-8, 129, 143, 144, 145, 154,
    158, 164, 165, 170, 171, 177, **188**
sandalwood 158

saw palmetto 135, **138,** 141, **188**
sciatica 70
septicaemia 130, 134
shepherd's purse **140,** 144, 145,
    147, 172, **188**
shingles 91, **92,** 93
side effects 11-12
sinusitis **110-11,** 112
sitz bath 147
skin 113-34
skin infections **130-1,** 134
skin ulcers 133
sleep aids 81, 82, 83, 85
slippery elm bark 18, 20, 49
sore throat 99, 102, **111**
splinters 24, **131**
sprains 69, **78-9**
stage fright **88-9**
stamina, mental and physical
    155-7
stomach ache 28, **64**
stomach cramps 70
stomach overacidity 47, 48, **65**
stomach ulcers 47, 66
stomach underacidity **64-5**
storing dried herbs 174
stress 38, 39, 48, 54, 81, 82, 84,
    86, **92-3,** 151, 154
stroke, recovery from 37
stye **131-2**
sunburn 114, 115, **132-3**
suppliers 15, 20, 167-8
sweating 139
swollen legs/feet 44
syrups 24, 178

tea tree 110, **118,** 120, 126, 131, 148,
    184, **188**
teas see infusions
thrush 137, 140, **147-8**
thuja 133
thyme 28, 61, **100,** 103, 104, 106,
    107, 112, **115,** 126, 128, 131, 132-3,
    137, 142, 147, 148, 164, 170, 171,
    178, 182, **188**
tinctures 21-2, 30
    for children 26-7
    concentrated 21
    dosage 25
    herb mixtures 31

    making 175-6
    standardised 21
    strengths 21, 25, 175-6
    taking 22
tisanes see infusions
tonsillitis 99, **111-12**
travelling abroad with herbs 9,
    180-4
turmeric 36, **74,** 78, 163, **188**

ulcerative colitis/Crohn's disease
    66
unhappiness 160
urethritis 136, 138, **141-2**
urinary and reproductive systems
    135-49
urine retention 141
urticaria (hives) 117, 133
uterine prolapse 140, **147**

vaginal discharge 140
valerian **39,** 42, **81,** 86-7, 89, 90,
    91, 92, 93, 108, **118, 137,** 146,
    147, 158, 171, 172, 182, **188**
varicose veins 34, 38, **44**
vervain **55,** 56, 59, 65, **86,** 88, 145,
    154, 158, 160, 161, 164, 165,
    172, **188**
vomiting 16, **65-6**

warts and verrucas **133**
well-being, enhancing 160-1
white deadnettle **140,** 148, 172,
    188
wild yam **74,** 77, **140-1,** 143, 144,
    145, 157, **188**
wildlife, attracting 19, 169
willow bark **70-1,** 75, 77, 182, **188**
wind, excess 51, 57, **59**
wintergreen **74,** 75, 78, 157, 171,
    188
witch hazel 44, **55-6,** 58, 120, 171,
    188
worm infestations 52, **66**
wounds see cuts and grazes

yarrow **34-5,** 40, 42, 43, 44, 125,
    137-8, 145, 146, 172, **188**
yellow dock 57, **119,** 120, 129, 172,
    188